# PERFECT HEALTH

## THE COMPLETE GUIDE FOR BODY & MIND

# Stress & Alternative Therapies

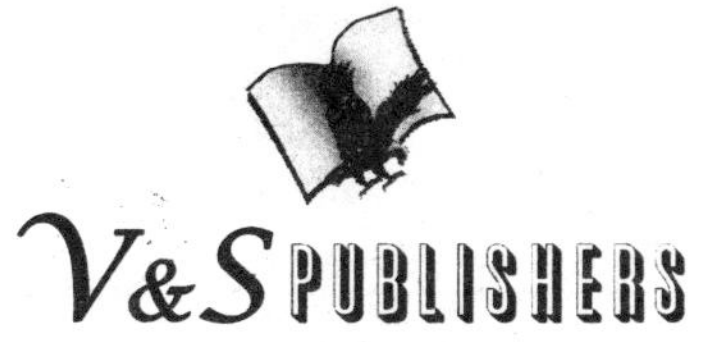

***Published by:***

F-2/16, Ansari Road, Daryaganj, New Delhi-110002
011-23240026, 011-23240027 • *Fax:* 011-23240028
*Email:* info@vspublishers.com • *Website:* www.vspublishers.com

**Branch : Hyderabad**
5-1-707/1, Brij Bhawan (Beside Central Bank of India Lane)
Bank Street, Koti, Hyderabad - 500 095.
040-24737290.
*E-mail:* vspublishershyd@gmail.com





ISBN 978-93-815883-9-0
**Edition 2014**



***Printed at :*** Param Offseters, Okhla, New Delhi-110020

# PUBLISHER'S NOTE

According to Francis Bacon, "A healthy body is the greatest chamber of soul; a sick one, its prison." But to maintain a healthy body one must not only follow the rules of moderate health living coupled with a state of moral relaxation exercising one's judgment in meeting the strains and stresses in life but must also understand the disease process, since a proper understanding of not only the health but also of the sickness is essential in maintaining a healthy being.

The present day stress of life produces harmful effects not only on different organs of the body but also on the psyche. There is no denying the fact that both the mind and body are so interlinked that their mutual interaction constitutes equal share in the maintenance of the normal human cycle.

To live a normal healthy life one has to live life and enjoy it. Life can't be a mathematical equation of do's and don't but, put in a judicious manner; the various intricacies of a healthy and diseased body must be well appreciated. If one can understand that the road to healthy living through a life of moderation in one's habit and attitudes towards life, the task becomes much easier.

To make the task easier we present to you *Perfect Health,* a set of four books.

**Book I:** Perfect Health: Body, Diet & Nutrition
**Book II:** Perfect Health: Fitness & Slimming
**Book III:** Perfect Health: Health Hazards & Cure
**Book IV:** Perfect Health: Stress & Alternative Therapies

This set of four books is not meant to create awareness about the physical well-being alone. There are many books doing that, already. Instead, all the four books are all about creating awareness that fitness of the mind and emotions is as important as the fitness of body. And unless one works at being fit in every way, one is not likely to find true health.

To many, this would seem an unattainable goal but it is not so. The effort required to work towards an integrated health and fitness regime is hardly any more difficult than trying to balance your social and spiritual life. Where there is a will, there is a way. And so with fitness.

*Perfect Health* provides a complete step-by-step program of mind body medicine tailored to individual needs. The result is a total plan, tailor-made for each individual, to reestablish the body's essential balance with nature; to strengthen the mind-body connection; and to use the power of quantum healing to transcend the ordinary limitations of disease and aging – in short, for achieving perfect health.

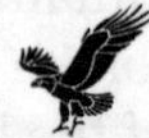

# CONTENTS

# SECTION 1

## STRESS

*Chapter* **1**

# STRESS AND WHAT CAUSES IT?

## Mind

There are times when we all need a physical and psychological boost to push us over the hump. This means that the mind has a great amount of hold on one's feeling of well-being. Which is why I guess the saying a *healthy mind, in a healthy body*, holds true.

Speaking of the interplay of healthy mind and healthy body, it is like speaking of self-development. For when the body is healthy, your mind automatically becomes free of worries and you can concentrate on more productive issues.

Among the low phases of natural living, one has to deal with one more factor that has made its appearance in the last few decades. It is stress I. If there is any, truly, global phenomenon, it is stress.

**STRESS** is an inescapable part of modern life. The good news is that stress isn't altogether bad news. In metered doses, it can be helpful...it can even make you better at what you do, and help give you the competitive edge.

Stress is an adaptive response. It's the body's reaction to an event that is seen as emotionally disturbing, disquieting, or threatening. When we perceive such an event, we experience what one stress researcher called the "fight or flight" response. To prepare for fighting or fleeing, the body increases its heart rate and blood pressure; more blood is then sent to your heart and muscles, and your respiration rate increases.

Our stress response is more likely triggered by overwhelming responsibilities at home or work, by loneliness, or by the fear of losing our jobs. Not only is uncontrolled stress harmful to our bodies in and of itself, but it can also lead to unwise behaviours such as alcohol and drug abuse, which place us at even greater risk, health wise. It can also jeopardize our relationships, by leading to emotional outbursts and, in some cases, physical violence.

The word 'stress' is taken from engineering jargon; in essence it means the deformation or change caused on a body by the internal forces that work on it. The maximum stress a body can withstand and still return to its normal state is known as its 'elastic limit'. This applies on people, too – an individual has his or her own elastic limit, both in terms of degree and type of stress. It is when the body is put under long-term stress that it can reach its snapping point; if it does the damage can be irreparable.

There are several major sources of stress:

- **Survival stress:** this may occur in cases where your survival or health is threatened, where you are put under pressure, or where you experience some unpleasant or challenging event. Here adrenaline is released in your body and you experience all the symptoms of your body preparing for 'fight or flight'.
- **Internally generated stress:** this can come from anxious worrying about events beyond your control, from a tense, hurried approach to life, or from relationship problems caused by your own behaviour. It can also come from an 'addiction' to and enjoyment of stress
- **Environmental and job stress:** here your living or working environment causes the stress. It may come from noise, crowding, pollution, untidiness, dirt or other distractions. Alternatively stress can come from events at work.
- **Fatigue and overwork:** here stress builds up over a long period. This can occur where you try to achieve too much in too little time, or where you are not using effective time management strategies.

Of all the stressors, the ones related to lifestyle and jobs are the most common. In fact, they form the bulk of stressors. Let us have a look at some of them, it will help you to identify these stressors and learn to deal with them.

## Lifestyle and Job Stress

Many of the stresses you experience may come from your job or lifestyle. These may include:

### Job related stressors:

- ❑ Too much or too little work
- ❑ Having to perform beyond your experience or perceived abilities
- ❑ Having to overcome unnecessary obstacles
- ❑ Time pressures and deadlines
- ❑ Keeping up with new developments
- ❑ Changes in procedures and policies
- ❑ Lack of relevant information, support and advice, lack of clear objectives, unclear expectations of your role from your boss or colleagues, responsibility for people, budgets or equipment.

### Career development stress:

- ❑ Under employment, non-promotion, frustration and boredom with current role
- ❑ Over-promotion beyond abilities
- ❑ Lack of a clear plan for career development
- ❑ Lack of opportunity
- ❑ Lack of job security

### Personal and family stress:

- ❑ Financial problems
- ❑ Relationship problems
- ❑ Ill-health
- ❑ Family changes such as birth, death, marriage or divorce.

## Stress Symptoms

Stress may manifest itself through various symptoms, which can be divided into three categories–

- ❑ Emotional
- ❑ Behavioural and
- ❑ Physical

## Emotional symptoms of stress

Stress causes many complaints and conditions. When one or more of the signs or symptoms occur frequently, or are more difficult to shrug off, it indicates that your stress level is becoming unacceptably high. And it is time to review your lifestyle and take steps to reduce stress.

- ❑ Worry or anxiety
- ❑ Confusion, and an inability to concentrate or make decisions
- ❑ Feeling ill
- ❑ Feeling out of control or overwhelmed by events

***Mood changes:***

- ❑ Depression
- ❑ Frustration
- ❑ Hostility
- ❑ Helplessness
- ❑ Impatience & irritability
- ❑ Restlessness
- ❑ Being more lethargic
- ❑ Difficulty in sleeping
- ❑ Drinking more alcohol and smoking more
- ❑ Changing eating habits
- ❑ Reduced sex drive
- ❑ Relying more on medication

## Behavioural symptoms of stress

Stress influences behaviour. Behavioural symptoms of long term stress are:

- ❑ Talking too fast or too loud
- ❑ Yawning
- ❑ Fiddling and twitching, nail biting, grinding teeth, drumming fingers, pacing, etc.

***Bad moods:***

- ❑ Being irritable
- ❑ Defensiveness
- ❑ Being critical
- ❑ Aggression

- ❑ Irrationality
- ❑ Overreaction and reacting emotionally

***Reduced personal effectiveness:***

- ❑ Being unreasonably negative
- ❑ Making less realistic judgements
- ❑ Being unable to concentrate and having difficulty making decisions
- ❑ Being more forgetful
- ❑ Making more mistakes
- ❑ Being more accident prone
- ❑ Changing work habits
- ❑ Increased absenteeism
- ❑ Neglect of personal appearance

These symptoms of stress should not be taken in isolation - other factors could cause them. However if you find yourself exhibiting or recognising a number of them, then it would be worth investigating stress management

## Physical symptoms of stress

The physical symptoms can be of two kinds – the **short-term symptoms** and the **long-term symptoms.**

### *Short term physical symptoms*

These mainly occur as your body adapts to perceived physical threat, and are caused by release of adrenaline. Although you may perceive these as unpleasant and negative, they are signs that your body is ready for the explosive action that assists survival or high performance:

- ❑ Faster heart beat
- ❑ Increased sweating
- ❑ Cool skin
- ❑ Cold hands and feet
- ❑ Feelings of nausea, or 'Butterflies in stomach'
- ❑ Rapid Breathing
- ❑ Tense Muscles
- ❑ Dry Mouth
- ❑ A desire to urinate
- ❑ Diarrhoea

### *Long term physical symptoms*

These occur where your body has been exposed to adrenaline over a long period. One of the ways adrenaline prepares you for action is by diverting resources to the muscles from the areas of the body, which carry out body maintenance. This means that if you are exposed to adrenaline for a sustained period, then your health may start to deteriorate. This may show up in several ways like:

- ❑ Change in appetite
- ❑ Frequent colds
- ❑ Asthma
- ❑ Back pain
- ❑ Digestive problems
- ❑ Headaches
- ❑ Skin eruptions
- ❑ Sexual disorders
- ❑ Aches and pains
- ❑ Feelings of intense and long-term tiredness

## Assessing Stress Levels

Emotional trauma caused by divorce, bereavement and moving house are stressful life events. Researchers discovered that our adaptability and ability to relax and cope with stress is damaged when we go through prolonged period of stressful life events. Some people find one particular life event more damaging than another; heredity, lifestyle and diet all affect an individual's response to stress.

Here are some life events and stress points connected with them:

| | |
|---|---|
| Death of a partner | 100 |
| Divorce | 73 |
| Separation from partner | 65 |
| Death of close family member | 63 |
| Injury or illness | 53 |
| Getting married | 50 |
| Termination of job | 47 |

| | |
|---|---|
| Pregnancy | 40 |
| Retirement | 45 |
| Ill health of a family member | 44 |
| Sexual difficulties | 39 |
| Major business or work changes | 39 |
| Change in financial state | 38 |
| Death of a friend | 37 |
| More arguments with partner | 35 |
| Change in responsibilities at work | 29 |
| Child leaves home | 29 |
| Trouble with in-laws | 29 |
| Outstanding personal achievement | 28 |
| Changes in living conditions | 25 |
| Trouble with boss or employer | 23 |
| Change in residence | 20 |
| Change in social activities | 18 |
| Change in sleeping habits | 16 |
| Change in eating habits | 15 |
| *Minor violations of the law | 11 |
| Individual stress levels can be worked out according to the above scale. | |
| **Score** | **Risk** |
| 100 Points | 10% increase of illness over the next 2 years. |
| 100-300 Points | 50% increase of illness over the next 2 years. |
| Above 300 Points | Dangerous risk of illness over the next 2 years. |
| *Source:* Rahe-Holmes lige change index. | |

## How can it be eliminated

A stress free existence is, perhaps, a mirage. The pressures of modern living ensure that stress is always lurking in the background. It can't be eliminated but one could try to control it.

Stress can be good and bad, depending on the type. Positive stress adds anticipation and excitement to life, and we all thrive under a certain amount of stress. Deadlines, competitions, confrontations, and even our frustrations and sorrows add depth and enrichment to our lives. Our goal is not to eliminate stress but to learn how to manage it and how to use it to help us. Insufficient stress acts as a depressant and may leave us feeling bored or dejected; on the other hand, excessive stress may leave us feeling "tied up in knots." What we need to do is find the optimal level of stress, which will individually motivate but not overwhelm each of us.

## What is optimal stress

There is no single level of stress that is optimal for all people. We are all individual creatures with unique requirements. As such, what is distressing to one may be a joy to another. And even when we agree that a particular event is distressing, we are likely to differ in our physiological and psychological responses to it. The person who loves to arbitrate disputes and moves from job site to job site would be stressed in a job, which was stable, and routine, whereas the person who thrives under stable conditions would very likely be stressed on a job when duties were highly varied. Also, our personal stress requirements and the amount which we can tolerate before we become distressed changes with our ages.

It has been found that most illness is related to unrelieved stress. If you are experiencing stress symptoms, you have gone beyond your optimal stress level; you need to reduce the stress in your life and/or improve your ability to manage it.

## Two Types of Personalities

Stress-prone personalities are classified as Type A and hardy personalities are said to belong to Type B. Type B personalities show better resistance to stress.

**Type A personalities** are disease prone and given to feelings of depression, anger, hostility and anxiety, which in turn makes them susceptible to asthma, headaches, ulcers, arthritis and heart disease, amongst others. Hostility is a significant factor associated with a greater risk of coronary heart disease in such individuals. Type A individuals have increased cortisol levels, which may interfere in the metabolism of lips and cholesterol and contribute to formation of fatty plaques in the arteries.

Such ultra stress-prone individuals tend to be hyper-responsive to stress. They ruminate or daydream about stressful events, cannot put stressors out of their mind and sometimes have nightmares about specific stressors.

**Type B personalities** display three characteristics – commitment, control and challenge. High on all three counts, hardy individuals exhibit feelings of meaningfulness in their work and relationships, a sense of being in control of events around them, and a tendency to interpret stressors as challenges that will be overcome.

## How to manage stress better

Identifying unrelieved stress and being aware of its effect on our lives is not sufficient for reducing its harmful effects. Just as there are many sources of stress, there are many possibilities for its management. However, all require work toward change: changing the source of stress and/or changing your reaction to it.

## How To Proceed

### Become aware of stressors

Notice your stress. Don't ignore it. Don't gloss over your problems. Determine what events stress you. What are you telling yourself about meaning of these events? Determine how your body responds to the stress. Do you become nervous or physically upset? If so, in what specific ways?

## Recognize change

Can you change your stressors by avoiding or eliminating them completely? Can you reduce their intensity (manage them over a period of time instead of on a daily or weekly basis)? Can you shorten your exposure to stress (take a break, leave the physical premises)?

Can you devote the time and energy necessary to making a change (goal setting, time management techniques, and delayed gratification strategies may be helpful here)?

## Reduce the intensity of emotional reactions to stress

The stress reaction is triggered by your perception of danger...physical danger and/or emotional danger. Are you viewing your stressors in exaggerated terms and/or taking a difficult situation and making it a disaster? Are you expecting to please everyone?

Are you overreacting and viewing things as absolutely critical and urgent? Do you feel you must always prevail in every situation? Work at adopting more moderate views; try to see the stress as something you can cope with rather than something that overpowers you. Try to temper your excess emotions. Put the situation in perspective. Do not labour on the negative aspects and the " what if" imagination.

## Learn to moderate physical reactions to stress

Slow, deep breathing will bring your heart rate and respiration back to normal.

Relaxation techniques can reduce muscle tension. Electronic biofeedback can help you gain voluntary control over such things as muscle tension, heart rate, and blood pressure.

Medications, when prescribed by a physician, can help in the short term in moderating your physical reactions. However, they alone are not the answer. Learning to moderate these reactions on your own is a preferable long-term solution.

## Build physical reserves

Exercise for cardiovascular fitness three to four times a week (moderate, prolonged rhythmic exercise is best, such as walking, swimming, cycling, or jogging).

- Eat well-balanced, nutritious meals.
- Maintain your ideal weight.
- Avoid nicotine, excessive caffeine, and other stimulants.
- Mix leisure with work. Take breaks and get away when you can.
- Get enough sleep. Be as consistent with your sleep schedule as possible.

## Maintain emotional reserves

Develop some mutually supportive friendships/ relationships. Pursue realistic goals, which are meaningful to you, rather than goals others have for you that you do not share. Expect some frustrations, failures, and sorrows. Always be kind and gentle with yourself—be a friend to yourself.

Chapter 2

# STRESSORS

## Ask yourself

- ❑ Are you a perfectionist?
- ❑ Do you feel a constant pressure to achieve?
- ❑ Do you criticize yourself when you're not perfect?
- ❑ Do you feel you haven't done enough no matter how hard you try?
- ❑ Do you give up pleasure in order to be the best in everything you do?
- ❑ Does your self-esteem depend on everyone else's opinion of you? Do you sometimes avoid assignments because you're afraid of disappointing your boss?
- ❑ Are you better at caring for others than caring for yourself?
- ❑ Do you keep most negative feelings inside to avoid displeasing others?

If the answer to all these questions is a 'yes', then you are a victim of stress.

## Helpful Techniques

Keep a record of stressful situations and rate the actual level of stress from O (most relaxed) to 10 (most stressed). As you begin to observe your levels of stress, you will notice that these levels are not constant.

You will find that stress levels increase when you are concentrating on your most alarming thoughts and bodily reactions, but stress levels fall when your attention turns away from these areas. This will show you that one way to reduce the level of stress in your life is to actively turn away from negative "stress building" thoughts and to concentrate on positive stress busting ways of thinking. Combating negative thoughts and replacing them with positive ones takes practice, but the results are worth it. Review the facts.

What is your evidence? Is there another way to view the situation? If not, what is the worst thing that could happen? You may have been concentrating on the worst possible, but by no means the most likely, outcome.

## Coping With Stress

The most common questions in magazines, doctor's clinics, helplines and social circles is –'how do I cope with my stress level'. There are dozens of remedies and ways but there are no magic cures. One has to deal with his/her stress in an individual and special manner. What works for one may not work for another? However, here are some very effective methods, which deal with almost every aspect of stress -

- Change your thinking
- Change your behaviour
- Change your lifestyle

### Change your thinking

- Practice reframing of thoughts
- Use the power of positive thinking
- Change your behaviour
- Be assertive
- Get organized/ learn the technique of time management
- Express your feelings (ventilate)
- Develop a strong sense of humour
- Pick up some hobby
- Change your lifestyle
- Healthy diet is the key to a healthy mind
- Exercise regularly
- Drink gallons of water
- Pet therapy is very effective
- Try meditation
- Deep breathing relieves stress
- Nature walks and imagery are extremely useful
- Practice the magic of hydrotherapy
- Indulge in soulful music therapy
- Grab enough sleep
- Make time for leisure

## Helpful Tips

### Stress control through positive thinking

Avoid negative thoughts of powerlessness, dejection, failure and despair. Chronic stress makes us vulnerable to negative suggestion. Learn to focus on positives.

### Get organized

One of the most common causes of stress is being disorganized at work or at home. Here are some tips to get organized. Keep a diary. Write lists of tasks to accomplish prioritise them and schedule when you will complete them.

Writing down objectives, duties and activities helps to make them more tangible and doable. Having a schedule also helps you provide the facts when your boss asks you to perform unreasonable tasks. They may have no idea that you are overwhelmed with work and the additional responsibilities cannot be accomplished unless something else goes. Again, prioritising tasks helps you to minimize the stressful situations.

### Make a list

So many projects, so little time. To beat stress, you have to learn to prioritise. At the start of each day, pick the single most important task to complete, and then finish it. If you're a person who makes to-do lists, never write one with more than five items. That way, you're more likely to get all the things done, and you'll feel a greater sense of accomplishment and control. Then you can go ahead and make a second five-item list. While you're at it, make a list of things that you can delegate to co-workers and family members.

### Learn to say 'no'

Sometimes you have to learn to draw the line. Stressed-out people often can't assert themselves. Instead of saying 'I don't want to do this' or 'I need some help,' they do it all themselves. Then they have even more to do."

Give your boss a choice. Give your boss a choice. Say 'I'd really like to take this on, but I can't do that without giving up something else. Which of these things would you like me to do?' Most bosses can take the hint. The same strategy works at home, with your spouse, children, relatives and friends.

If you have trouble-saying 'no', start small. Tell your hubby to make his own sandwich. Or tell your daughter to find another ride home from volleyball practice. Pad your schedule. Realize that nearly everything will take longer than you anticipate. By allotting yourself enough time to accomplish a task, you cut back on anxiety. In general, if meeting deadlines is a problem, always give yourself 20 percent more time than you think you need to do the task.

## Time Management

Look at the way you do things. Are you a perfectionist? If so, try to decide which tasks truly require meticulous attention to detail and which can be done casually.

Make a realistic list of what you need to accomplish in a given day, with the most important things at the top. Tackle them one at a time, and don't start a second until you have finished the first. Plan your day to include work breaks which physically or mentally take you away from the office, Try not to bring office work home. When you have several things to accomplish, set priorities and postpone less important tasks. Learn to delegate matters that cannot be put off. Deal with concerns on a day-at-a-time basis. Control the timing of stressful events. Try not to make major decisions when you are overtired or anxious.

## Ventilation

People who keep things for themselves without sharing with their friends or loved ones carry a considerable and unnecessary burden. Share your problems and concern with others. Develop a support system of relatives, colleagues or friends to talk to when you are upset or worried. When you are frustrated write it down. After you have vent the frustration, destroy the writing so that it is forgotten. Re-reading the journal will reawaken the frustration and anger. So, do not keep it.

Seek social support. Studies have shown that close, positive relationships with others facilitate good health and morale. One reason for this is that support from family and friends serves as a buffer to cushion the impact of stressful events. Talking out problems and expressing tensions can be incredibly helpful.

## Laughter therapy

Humour is a wonderful stress-reducer and antidote to upsets. It is clinically proven to be effective in combating stress, although the exact mechanism is not known. Experts say a good laugh relaxes tense muscles, speeds more oxygen into your system and lowers your blood pressure. So tune into your favourite sitcom on television. Read a funny book. Call a friend and chuckle for a few minutes. It even helps to force a laugh once in a while. You'll find your stress melting away almost instantly.

Laughter therapy is turning out to be the most successful stress buster. Laughter stimulates the immune system, off-setting the immunosuppressive effects of stress.

We know that, during stress, the adrenal gland releases corticosteroids (quickly converted to cortisol in the blood stream) and that elevated levels of these have an immuno-suppressive effect. Laughter can lower cortisol levels and thereby protect our immune system.

**The emotions and moods we experience directly affect our immune system.** A sense of humour allows us to perceive and appreciate the incongruities of life and provides moments of joy and delight. These positive emotions can create neurochemical changes that will buffer the immunosuppressive effects of stress.

A belly laugh is really good for you. It relieves muscular tension, improves breathing, and regulates the heartbeat. Watch comedy shows and laugh. Or attend comedy shows. Read comics or humour books. Share funny episodes with your spouse so that both can relieve stress as well improve communication between the two of you.

## An anti-stress diet

A well balanced diet is crucial in preserving health and helping to reduce stress. Certain foods and drinks act as powerful stimulants to the body and hence are a direct cause of stress. Stress affects the body's ability to handle various kinds of foods because it causes a sudden constriction of the blood vessels. This raises blood pressure and reduces the amount of blood flowing to the stomach and intestines. The flow of enzymes is slowed down so much of the food that is eaten is poorly digested. Instead of being broken down properly, it ferments in the intestine causing gas and distension. Here are some tips on following an anti-stress diet-

## Foods to Control

### Sodium

Cut down on table salt and other sources of sodium because of their link with high blood pressure.

### Caffeine

This is found in coffee, tea, chocolate, coke, etc. It causes the release of adrenaline, thus increasing the level of stress. When taken in moderation, coffee can increase your alertness, increased activity in the muscles, nervous system and heart. Consuming too much caffeine has the same effect as long-term stress. It is suggested that there is a link between caffeine intake and high blood pressure and high cholesterol levels.

Be careful in reducing the coffee or caffeine consumption. Cutting it off abruptly can result in your experiencing withdrawal symptoms. Reduce the consumption slowly over a period of time.

### Alcohol

Like caffeine, taken in moderation, alcohol is a very useful drug. It has been shown to benefit cardiovascular system. Alcohol is a number one cause of stress. The irony of the situation is that most people take to drinking as way to combat stress. But, in actuality, they make it worse by consuming alcohol. Alcohol and stress, in combination, is quite deadly.

Alcohol stimulates the secretion of adrenaline resulting in the problems such as nervous tension, irritability and insomnia. Excess alcohol will increase the fat deposits in the heart and decrease the immune function. Alcohol also limits the ability of the liver to remove toxins from the body. During stress, the body produces several toxins such as hormones. In the absence of its filtering by the liver, these toxins continue to circulate through the body resulting in serious damage.

### Smoking

Many people use cigarettes as a coping mechanism. In the short term, smoking seems to relieve stress. But in the long term smoking is very harmful. Its disadvantages far outweigh its short-term benefits. Cigarette smoking is shown to be responsible for a variety of cancers, hypertension, respiratory illness and heart disease.

## Foods Priority

### Food high in fibre

Stress result in cramps and constipation. Eat more fibre to keep your digestive system moving. Your meal should provide at least 25 grams of fibre per day. Fruits, vegetables and grains are excellent sources of fibre. For breakfast, eat whole fruits instead of just juice, and whole-grain cereals and fibre-fortified muffins.

### Vegetables

Your brain's production of serotonin is sensitive to your diet. Eating more vegetables can increase your brain's serotonin production. This increase is due to improved absorption of the amino acid L-Tryptophan. (Vegetables contain the natural, safe, form of L Tryptophan). Meats contain natural L-Tryptophan also, but when you eat meat, the L-Tryptophan has to compete with so many other amino acids for absorption that the L-Tryptophan loses out.

### Water

Drink nothing less than 8-10 glasses of this precious liquid. It helps to flush waste products out of the body.

### Vitamins and minerals

Eat foods rich in potassium like oranges and bananas. Potassium is essential for maintaining the balance of minerals within body fluids and plays a key role in muscle contraction.

Get a lot of calcium into the system, as you tend to lose it when you are stressed. Try to have at least two glasses of skimmed milk every day.

**Vitamin C** is an important factor, as it keeps the walls of the capillaries flexible. The blood vessels constrict at the first sign of stress, and this results in the depletion of vitamin C in the body.

**Vitamin B** serves as a catalyst in the production of energy, and in the metabolism of protein and fats. It is also necessary for the central nervous system. In conditions of stress, supplements are advisable. Increase the intake of green leafy vegetables, eggs, milk, whole grains and yeast.

### Fruits

Include fruits like bananas, apples, apricots, cherries, grape fruit, melons, oranges, peaches, pears, pineapple, plums etc. They are rich in potassium and low in sodium.

## Stress and Exercise

Research has shown that physical exercise is the best tension reliever. It is a very important remedy for stress. Nothing eases stress more than exercise.

Physically, exercise improves your cardiovascular functions by strengthening and enlarging the heart, causing greater elasticity of the blood vessels, increasing oxygen throughout your body, and lowering levels of fats such as cholesterol and triglycerides. All of this, of course, means less chance of developing heart conditions, strokes, or high blood pressure.

Exercise improves mood by producing positive biochemical changes in the body and brain. Regular exercise reduces the amount of adrenal hormones your body releases in response to stress. Exercise, therefore, will keep your body functioning properly and will keep you feeling both relaxed, refreshed and promote deep, restful sleep.

Exercise has another beneficial effect. Most people, when exercising, do not worry. They are actually resting the nerve cells in the brain that worry, giving those cells time to renew themselves, so they can function normally the next time they are needed. Dancing, listening to music, reading, working on a craft, playing a musical instrument, meditation, self-relaxation, and biofeedback also relieve stress. Any activity, which concentrates your attention on a subject other than life's problems, will help rest your mind. This allows the brain to renew itself.

## Exercise should be done at least five days each week

The human body craves consistency and can make adjustments to long-term demands placed upon it. If you exercise three times per week, it will have a conditioning effect on your heart, but the heart is not the only thing that needs to perform efficiently during exercise. The other organs and muscle tissues will respond much differently to five days in a row. For five days in a row, the body continues to receive the message that it needs to perform efficiently in order to keep up. It adjusts to meet the demand and the result is efficient operation of the whole system, all the time, even on the two days you don't exercise.

Most people gain weight due to stress and not because of increased food intake or reduction in activity levels. Combining regular, vigorous exercise along with eliminating stress can bring about a significant weight reduction.

## Toughies vs Weaklings

At a simple level it may appear that a measure of 'toughness' is how well you keep on going under extreme stress. This is simplistic. It is certainly possible to be self-indulgent and use stress as an excuse for not pushing yourself hard enough. It is, however, also far too easy to let yourself be pushed to a level where your work, and physical and mental health start to suffer. The strongest and most flexible position is to actively manage your levels of stress and fatigue so that you are able to produce high quality work over a long period, reliably.

High performance in your job may require continued hard work in the face of high levels of sustained stress. If this is the case, it is essential that you learn to pay attention to your feelings. This ensures that you know when to relax, slacken off for a short period, get more sleep, or implement stress management strategies. If you do not take feelings of tiredness, upset or discontent seriously, then you may face failure, burn-out or breakdown. As well as paying attention to your own stress levels, it may be worth paying attention to the stress under which people around you operate. If you are a manager seeking to improve productivity, then failing to monitor stress may mean that you drive employees into depression or burn-out. If this is a danger, then reduce stress for long enough for them to recover, and then reconsider the pace you are setting.

## What can Happen if Stress gets Out of Control

Where you are under excessive levels of short-term stress, then you may find that your performance goes to pieces. Afterwards, however, you will be able to treat this as a learning experience and can adopt stress management strategies to avoid the problem in the future.

The effects of long-term stress going out of control can be much more severe. If you do not take action to control it, this can lead to:

- ❑ Hurry Sickness
- ❑ Burn Out, or Breakdown

## Hurry Sickness

A particularly unpleasant source of stress comes from 'Hurry Sickness'.

Here you can get into a vicious circle of stress, which causes you to hurry jobs and do them badly. This under-performance causes feelings of frustration and failure, which causes more stress, which causes more hurry and less success, and so on. Stress-creating behaviour can compound this, as can an inability to relax at home or on holiday. If you do not manage long-term stress effectively, it can lead to long-term fatigue, failure and one of the forms of physical or mental ill health.

Very often you can eliminate this sort of overload by effective use of time management skills, particularly by learning how to prioritise effectively. You can neutralise the associated stress by effective use of stress management techniques.

## Burn-Out Syndrome

More and more people are talking about a phenomenon called 'Burn-Out', these days. Young executives, software personnel and employees in media are especially prone to this problem. Burn-out is nothing but excessive stress exposure for a consistently long period. Earlier it was known as a 'Breakdown' which simply meant a break down of the human engine.

A boss who demands more and more and is never satisfied. A failing relationship that doesn't respond to anything you do. Children who are too demanding or disappointing, nagging spouses, all can lead to a breakdown.

All of these things tax the stress-coping resources and eventually, no matter how skilled your coping ability - you burn out. If coping skills are poor the burn-out happens sooner than if coping skills are good. At some point, in a high-pressure environment, coping -demands will exceed coping- skills, the ability to handle stress deteriorates, and burn-out occurs. It's analogous to driving a car. Driving a car at very fast speeds, for long periods of time, will burn out an engine. Trying to handle too much, all the time is the human equivalent.

## What is Burn-Out?

With increasing stress, coping skills begin to deteriorate. As coping skills deteriorate, vulnerability to stress multiplies and a vicious cycle ensues. It can result in failing mental and physical health, and premature death. To protect yourself, learn to recognize the early warning signs of coping burn-out and take immediate action.

## Recognising a Burn-Out

Some of the common symptoms of stress that may indicate you are approaching or already experiencing coping burn-out from too much stress are given below:

### Depression

Depression is both caused by stress and worsened by stress. If at least three or more of these symptoms have occurred over a period of the last two years, or have recurred episodically, see a psychotherapist for further evaluation.

Here are the symptoms to monitor.

- ❑ Insomnia (trouble sleeping) or hypersomnia (excessive sleeping).
- ❑ Low energy level or chronic tiredness.
- ❑ Feelings of inadequacy, loss of self-esteem, or self-depreciation.
- ❑ Decreased effectiveness or productivity at school, work, or home.
- ❑ Decreased attention, concentration, or ability to think clearly.
- ❑ Social withdrawal.
- ❑ Loss of interest in, or enjoyment of, activities, which normally produce pleasure.
- ❑ Irritability or excessive anger.
- ❑ Inability to respond with expressed pleasure to praise or rewards.
- ❑ Less active or talkative than usual, or feeling slowed down or restless.
- ❑ Pessimistic attitude toward the future, brooding about past events, or feeling sorry for oneself.
- ❑ Tearfulness or crying.
- ❑ Recurrent thoughts of death or suicide.

## Anxiety

Anxiety is the mind's natural response to an unknown, but anticipated danger. When no effective response to the anticipated danger is possible, or known, anxiety itself becomes the danger since it leads to physical debilitation and psychological immobilization. An evaluation by a psychotherapist is recommended when there are symptoms from the following four categories.

1. **Motor tension:** shakiness, jitteriness, jumpiness, trembling, tension, muscle aches, fatigability, inability to relax, eyelid twitch, furrowed brow, strained face, fidgeting, restlessness, being easily startled.
2. **Autonomic hyperactivity:** sweating, heart pounding or racing, cold, clammy hands, dry mouth, dizziness, light-headedness, paresthesias (tingling in hands or feet), upset stomach, hot or cold spells, frequent urination, diarrhoea, discomfort in the pit of the stomach, lump in the throat, flushing, pallor, high resting pulse and respiration rate.
3. **Apprehensive expectation:** anxiety, worry, fear, obsessive thinking, and anticipation of misfortune to self or others.
4. **Vigilance and scanning:** hyper-attentiveness resulting in distractibility, difficulty in concentrating, insomnia, feeling "on edge," irritability, impatience.

## Insomnia

Insomnia is characterized by; a) the inability to fall asleep, or, b) waking and not being able to go back to sleep.

Insomnia can be a symptom of anxiety and depression as well as excessive stress. Periodic insomnia is not abnormal and, while usually associated with excitement or concern (both are types of stress), it commonly goes away when the stressor is removed. However, chronic (long duration or frequent recurrence) insomnia is a danger sign and indicates excessive stress.

## Pain in the Back or Neck

The symptom of pain in either of these regions may be related to unconsciously tensing these muscles in a stressful situation. When chronically tensed they may become painful. Declaring that a job or supervisor is "a pain in the neck" may be literally true.

## Appetite Disturbance

Overeating or under-eating can be responses to stress. Under-eating results from a loss of appetite owing to excessive rumination (repetitious thinking on the same subject) and concern. Overeating is prevalent because overeating causes large amounts of blood to be diverted to the stomach and intestines to facilitate digestion. This reduces blood flow to the brain causing a slight tranquillising effect. Since eating tends to relax a person, people under stress tend to eat more. It's also a form of self-nurturing, with undesirable side effects. Gaining or losing weight unintentionally may be signs of excessive stress.

## Increased Smoking

The repetitious, ritual-like behaviour each smoker displays in smoking acts as a temporary tension reducer. Rituals bind anxiety and can be useful in dealing with tension. However, when the ritual is associated with behaviours having health-damaging side effects the potential health hazard overshadows any benefit. Large amounts of nicotine also serve to depress the central nervous system creating a sense of relaxation. Ironically, the overall effect is to elevate blood pressure, cholesterol, and noradrenaline. All of these are physical stressors endangering health. Therefore, the more you smoke, the more stressed you are; so you smoke more which creates more stress.... etc., etc. - a true Catch 22 situation. Get the picture?

## Increased Alcohol Consumption

Alcohol is an effective central nervous system depressant. It results in increased muscle relaxation and clouded thinking, which reduces mental tension. Precisely because it works so well it is a major danger during stressful periods. The potential for alcoholism, and alcohol abuse during periods of excessive stress demands proper vigilance and control.

## Abuse of Drugs

Excess stress produces an intense desire for the temporary escape provided by drugs. Both, stimulants (such as cocaine and amphetamines) and depressants (such as tranquillisers, opiates, barbiturates, and marijuana), serve as escape mechanisms and have a high potential for addiction and abuse. The temporary benefit is disproportionately low compared to the long-term damage associated with drug use and abuse.

## Increased Caffeine Intake

Increased intake of caffeine may be an indicator of coping burn-out. Caffeine serves two purposes in countering stress. The stimulant effect counteracts the lethargy from depression and the ritualistic activity of consumption reduces tension. Unfortunately, caffeine is also a physiological stressor. The average cup contains 100-150 milligrams of caffeine. As little as 250 milligrams of caffeine has been implicated in nervousness, insomnia, headaches, sweaty palms, and ulcers.

Following is a more specific list of symptoms, which have all been proven to be stress-related. Many of these symptoms may be caused by organic illnesses, but they are also symptoms of excessive stress. If you discover that you are answering a 'yes' to most of these pointers, it is time to visit your doctor and have a heart-to-heart chat with him.

- ❑ General irritability, hyper excitation, or depression.
- ❑ Pounding of the heart (high blood pressure symptom).
- ❑ Dryness of the throat and mouth.
- ❑ Impulsive behaviour, emotional instability.
- ❑ The overpowering urge to cry, or run and hide.
- ❑ Inability to concentrate, flight of thoughts, and general disorientation.
- ❑ Feelings of unreality, weakness, or dizziness. Predilection to become fatigued, and loss of the "joie de vivre" (the joy of life).
- ❑ "Floating anxiety," a generalized sense of apprehension without a focus.

- ❑ Emotional tension and alertness; a feeling of being "keyed up." Trembling, and nervous tics (involuntary muscle twitches, usually in the facial area).
- ❑ Tendency to become easily startled by inconsequential stimuli.
- ❑ High pitched, nervous laughter.
- ❑ Stuttering, and other speech difficulties.
- ❑ Bruxism (grinding the teeth, especially at night).
- ❑ Insomnia.
- ❑ Hyper motility; excessive activity in the stomach and intestines.
- ❑ Excessive sweating without physical exertion.
- ❑ The frequent need to urinate.
- ❑ Diarrhoea, indigestion, queasiness in the stomach, and vomiting.
- ❑ Migraine headaches.
- ❑ Premenstrual tension or missed menstrual cycles.
- ❑ Pain in the neck or lower back.
- ❑ Loss of appetite or compulsive eating.
- ❑ Increased smoking.
- ❑ Increased use of legally prescribed drugs, such as tranquillisers or stimulants.
- ❑ Alcohol and drug abuse or addiction.
- ❑ Nightmares.
- ❑ Psychosis.
- ❑ Accident proneness.

*Chapter* **3**

# ANXIETY, DEPRESSION, SLEEP AND INSOMNIA

Human life brings with it stresses and strains that are bound to make us unhappy. Loved ones die, jobs are lost, marriages or love affairs break up, and families quarrel among themselves. To be unmoved by these events is not possible. Confusion arises, however, because the word 'depression' is used in two different ways. Its most normal use is among ordinary people to cover ordinary feelings. People say they are depressed when they mean that they are feeling unhappy, down, miserable or gloomy. Most of us feel mildly depressed after an illness, or when we are tired, sometimes even when we are not able to pinpoint any reason. Women sometimes, find that depression is a part of pre-menstrual tension.

The word 'depression' is also used to cover something much more severe which makes the person ill with mental suffering. Severe depression can be triggered off by head injuries or concussion, some infections, operations on valued parts of the body – like having a leg amputated, hormonal changes, epilepsy, old age and the aftermath of a non-fatal stroke or thrombosis.

## ANXIETY

Anxiety is a term used by experts to mean the same as fear or worry. Sigmund Freud, the founder of psychoanalysis, showed that anxiety is a fundamental emotion that influences our lives from earliest childhood. People with neuroses frequently complain of excessive anxiety.

Anxiety occurs where you are concerned that circumstances are out of control. In some cases being anxious and worrying over a problem may generate a solution.

Normally it will just result in negative thinking. There are five main unrealistic desires or beliefs that cause anxiety:

- The desire always to have the love and admiration of all people important to you. This is unrealistic because you have no control over other people's minds. They can have bad days, see things in odd ways, make mistakes or can be plain disagreeable and awkward.
- The desire to be thoroughly competent at all times. This is unrealistic because you only achieve competence at a new level by making mistakes. Everybody has bad days and everybody makes mistakes.
- The belief that external factors cause all misfortune. Often negative events can be caused by your own negative attitudes. Similarly your own negative attitudes can cause you to view neutral events negatively. Someone else might find something positive in something you view as a problem. The desire that events should always turn out the way that you want them to, and that people should always do what you want. Other people have their own agendas and do what they want to do.
- The belief that past bad experience will inevitably control what will happen in the future. You can very often improve or change things if you try hard enough or look at things in a different way.

To be able to control these beliefs means to have a grip over anxiety.

## DEPRESSION

There is another ailment that is growing by leaps and bound in the modern era. This malady is very real and happens to many people. It is known as depression. For long, most doctors discarded it as a figment of imagination but in the recent past, a lot of studies and research have gone into this phenomenon and doctors are taking it very seriously.

### Symptoms

Major depression and anxiety problems share many symptoms. Some of the common symptoms shared by major depression and anxiety include unrealistic apprehension, fears, and worry; physical symptoms (headaches, irritable bowel syndrome, etc.); agitation; irritability; chronic fatigue; insomnia; or panic attacks. In fact, most depressed individuals—two out of three—also have anxiety symptoms.

- ❑ Psychotherapy and cognitive therapy can help treat depression with anxiety.
- ❑ About 80% of depressed individuals suffer psychological anxiety symptoms such as unrealistic apprehension, fears, and worries; agitation; irritability; or panic attacks.
- ❑ Some 60% of people with depression have anxiety-related physical symptoms like headaches, irritable bowel syndrome, chronic fatigue, and chronic pain, among others.
- ❑ Approximately 65% of depression sufferers experience sleeps disturbances.
- ❑ About 20% feel agitated.
- ❑ Some 25% have phobia.
- ❑ Approximately 17% report generalized anxiety symptoms.
- ❑ And 10% suffer panic attacks. In those with both depression and anxiety, the depression tends to strike earlier in life, tends be more severe, more chronic, more debilitating, and harder to treat successfully. Anxiety also increases depressed individuals' risk of suicide. For authenticity of the above figures, source must be given.

## Mild Depression

Tragic life events like bereavement, marriage failure, or job-loss can set off a mild depression. Society acknowledges that it is normal to feel unhappy after such events.

The normal reaction to a tragic event like a death is shock, and a kind of numbness. A great sense of loss clouds the mind. The next stage is often anger. The bereaved person is angry that the loved one has been taken away and may experience feelings of unfairness or anger against people who have not suffered such a loss. Sometimes denial sets in and the bereft person refuses to believe what has happened.

Finally, these painful feelings are superseded by feelings of acceptance and letting go. The anger burns itself out, and the person comes to terms with the loss. Then the stage is set for a return to normal living. Friends and relatives are usually helpful and sympathetic to somebody whose depression has a fairly obvious cause. This kind of depression can continue for quite some time, sometimes, up to two years.

## Severe Depression

This kind of depression is marked by its persistence and its acute painfulness for the sufferer.

Symptoms include guilt and a feeling of unworthiness, a loss of confidence, inability to concentrate, indecisiveness about even minor decisions like what to wear or eat, poor memory, agitation and anxiety, weeping, suicidal thoughts, irritability, fear of being alone, hopelessness, extreme weakness, tiredness and lethargy, delusions, fears about death, slowness of thought, loss of sexual desire, reduced appetite, insomnia and waking in the early hours of the morning, feeling worse in the morning and getting better in the day, loss of interest in life, self neglect, a preoccupation with bodily symptoms and bodily functions.

People who feel like this constantly, need professional help.

# SLEEP

Few things are more important than a good night's sleep. After a good sleep you are much more alert and capable of working or enjoying yourself to your full capacity. Lack of sleep makes a person slower and duller. During sleep, the body is busy repairing itself. Growth hormones pour into the body and stimulate the various tissues and organs of the body to repair themselves and grow. This is one reason why growing children need more sleep than adults. Even the brain is growing and repairing itself during sleep, and while doing this the blood supply to the brain increases and a person goes through a more wakeful period of dreaming sleep. Good sleep is essential for this process of bodily renewal, and if a person does not catch up on the lost sleep, he loses the ability to concentrate and to deal with the simplest of the problems.

There are two kinds of sleep. We start the night with deep sleep, but after one and a half to two hours we experience lighter dreaming-sleep, when our eyes make rapid movements and our electric brain waves are faster than in ordinary sleep. Psychologists call the period as 'rapid eye movement' sleep. These periods of dreaming-sleep occur about every one and a half hours during the night.

Many people suffer from the inability to sleep due to various factors, of which stress and depression rate the highest. People who suffer from depression often find it extremely difficult to sleep. A person who is depressed often feels worst in the morning and wakes up at 2 a.m. and again at 4 a.m. with the mind racing. Consequentially, such a person does not have the normal energy and is unable to do the normal tasks of life.

The inability to sleep is known as insomnia.

## INSOMNIA

Insomnia is the perception or complaint of inadequate or poor-quality sleep because of one or more of the following:

- ❑ Difficulty in falling asleep
- ❑ Waking up frequently during the night with difficulty returning to sleep
- ❑ Waking up too early in the morning
- ❑ Unrefreshing sleep

Individuals vary normally in their need for, and their satisfaction with, sleep. Insomnia may cause problems during the day, such as tiredness, a lack of energy, difficulty concentrating, and irritability. Insomnia can be classified as transient (short term), intermittent (on and off), and chronic (constant). Insomnia lasting from a single night to a few weeks is referred to as transient. If episodes of transient insomnia occur from time to time, the insomnia is said to be intermittent. Insomnia is considered to be chronic if it occurs on most nights and lasts a month or more.

## What causes it?

Certain conditions seem to make individuals more likely to experience insomnia. Examples of these conditions include:

- ❑ Advanced age (insomnia occurs more frequently in those over the age 60)
- ❑ Female gender
- ❑ A history of depression

If other conditions (such as stress, anxiety, a medical problem, or the use of certain medications) occur along with the above conditions, insomnia is more likely. There are many causes of insomnia. Transient and intermittent insomnia generally occur in people who are temporarily experiencing one or more of the following:

- ❑ Stress
- ❑ Environmental noise
- ❑ Extreme temperatures
- ❑ Change in the surrounding environment
- ❑ Sleep/wake schedule problems such as those due to jet lag
- ❑ Medication side effects

Chronic insomnia is more complex and often results from a combination of factors, including underlying physical or mental disorders. One of the most common causes of chronic insomnia is depression. Other underlying causes include arthritis, kidney disease, heart failure, asthma, sleep apnoea, narcolepsy, restless legs syndrome, Parkinson's disease, and hyperthyroidism. However, chronic insomnia may also be due to behavioural factors, including the misuse of caffeine, alcohol, or other substances; disrupted sleep/wake cycles as may occur with shift work or other night time activity schedules; and chronic stress.

In addition, the following behaviours have been shown to perpetuate insomnia:

- ❑ Expecting to have difficulty in sleeping and worrying about it
- ❑ Ingesting excessive amounts of caffeine
- ❑ Drinking alcohol before bedtime
- ❑ Smoking cigarettes before bedtime

- Excessive napping in the afternoon or evening
- Irregular or continually disrupted sleep/wake schedules

These behaviours may prolong existing insomnia, and they can also be responsible for causing the sleeping problem in the first place. Stopping these behaviours may eliminate the insomnia altogether.

## Who gets insomnia

Insomnia is found in males and females of all age groups, although it seems to be more common in females (especially after menopause) and in the elderly. The ability to sleep, rather than the need for sleep, appears to decrease with advancing age.

## Diagnosis

People with insomnia are evaluated with the help of a medical history and a sleep history. The sleep history may be obtained from a sleep diary filled out by the patient or by an interview with the patient's bed partner concerning the quantity and quality of the patient's sleep.

## Treatment

Transient and intermittent insomnia may not require treatment since episodes last only a few days at a time. For example, if insomnia is due to a temporary change in the sleep/wake schedule, as with jet lag, the person's biological clock will often get back to normal on its own. However, for some people who experience daytime sleepiness and impaired performance as a result of transient insomnia, the use of short-acting sleeping pills may improve sleep and next-day alertness. As with all drugs, there are potential side effects. The use of over-the-counter sleep medicines is not usually recommended for the treatment of insomnia.

### Treatment for chronic insomnia consists of:

- Diagnosing and treating underlying medical or psychological problems.

- Identifying behaviours that may worsen insomnia and stopping (or reducing) them.
- Possibly using sleeping pills, although the long-term use of sleeping pills for chronic insomnia is not advisable. A patient taking any sleeping pill should be under the supervision of a physician to closely evaluate effectiveness and minimize side effects. In general, these drugs are prescribed at the lowest dose and for the shortest duration needed to relieve the sleep-related symptoms. For some of these medicines, the dose must be gradually lowered as the medicine is discontinued because, if stopped abruptly, it can cause insomnia to occur again, for a night or two.
- Trying behavioural techniques to improve sleep, such as relaxation therapy, sleep restriction therapy, and reconditioning.

  **Relaxation therapy** - There are specific and effective techniques that can reduce or eliminate anxiety and body tension. As a result, the person's mind is able to stop "racing," the muscles can relax, and restful sleep can occur. It usually takes much practice to learn these techniques and to achieve effective relaxation.

  **Sleep restriction** - Some people suffering from insomnia spend too much time in bed unsuccessfully trying to sleep. They may benefit from a sleep restriction program that at first allows only a few hours of sleep during the night. Gradually the time is increased until a more normal night's sleep is achieved.

  **Reconditioning** – Another treatment that may help some people with insomnia is to recondition them to associate the bed and bedtime with sleep. For most people, this means not using their beds for any activities other than sleep and sex. As part of the reconditioning process, the person is usually advised to go to bed only when sleepy. If unable to fall asleep, the person is told to get up, stay up until sleepy, and then return to bed. Throughout this process, the person should avoid naps and wake up and go to bed at the same time, each day. Eventually the person's body will be conditioned to associate the bed and bedtime with sleep.

## Smart sleeping tips

- ❑ Maintain a regular sleep-wake pattern. Go to bed and wake up at the same times each day, including the weekend. Get up before sunrise because the early morning sunlight is best at resetting your biological clock.
- ❑ Don't exercise strenuously within two to three hours of retiring. Exercising early in the day helps you sleep, but exercising too close to bed keeps you awake.
- ❑ Don't eat a large meal within one to two hours of going to bed. Major digestive efforts can keep you up.
- ❑ Have a light snack before bed. A little bit of food before bed can help you sleep.
- ❑ Adopt bedtime rituals. Read for a while. Change into pyjamas. Brush your teeth. Lock your doors. Turn out your lights. Rituals help ease you into sleep.
- ❑ Turn down your thermostat. Cool temperatures help induce sleep.
- ❑ Don't nap during the day. Napping can interfere with night sleep.
- ❑ Limit your caffeine consumption. Drink less regular coffee. Caffeine can also be found in tea, colas, cocoa, chocolate, and many over-the-counter drugs (read labels and ask your pharmacist). Avoid caffeinated drinks eight hours prior to sleep.
- ❑ Avoid shift work. If possible, work from 9 to 5 or a schedule close to it. Working afternoons (4 to midnight) and nights (midnight to 8) disrupts sleep. The most sleep-disrupting schedule is a rotating shift work like alternating periods of day, afternoon, and night work.
- ❑ In addition, several antidepressant medications may disrupt sleep. If you take any of these medications and suffer sleep disturbances, you may not be aware of them. They may cause "micro-awakenings," momentary rousing during sleep, which you don't even realise, is happening.

- So how can you tell if your antidepressant is causing sleep disturbances? One tip-off is daytime drowsiness. If you have this, discuss it with your doctor. Dose adjustment may resolve the problem. If not, you might be able to switch to a medication not associated with sleep problems.
- Relax and unwind.
- Relaxation techniques calm you and let you forget your stresses for a while. Yoga or meditation often does the trick, as does massage or even a nice, warm bubble bath. Lovemaking is also a natural relaxant that can be quite effective before bedtime!

## Breath Yourself to Sleep

A cup of warm chamomile tea, followed by the yogic meditation posture (padmasana), is a great way to clear your mind and prepare for sleep.

### To get started:

- Sit in a comfortable cross-legged position. If you have muscle or joint pain, you can sit on a firm chair, with your feet flat on the floor. You can also sit on the edge of your bed. Hold your back erect, chest pulled up and forward. Relax your shoulders, but try not to slouch.
- If you're seated on a bed or chair, rest your hands palms down on your thighs. If you're seated on the floor, you can rest your hands comfortably on your thighs, palm-side up, thumb and index fingers touching. You can also cradle them in front of you, one on top of the other in your lap.
- Your chin should be parallel with the floor. Soften your facial muscles and let your mouth open slightly. Close your eyes.
- Slowly, breathe in deeply through your nose to the count of five. Hold the breath for five counts. Exhale slowly through your nose, counting to five. You want to feel your stomach muscles contract and your chest

expand on the inhalation. On the exhalation, use your stomach muscles to press out all of the air.

Repeat this posture for six to eight breaths.

## Relax Yourself to Sleep

Here is a modified yoga relaxation posture (shavasana) that you can do in your bed – you'll be right where you want to be when you nod off.

### To get started:

- ❑ In bed, lie on your back with your legs comfortably far apart, feet turned out. Shift your arms away from your body, place your hands palm side up, fingers slightly curved. Close your eyes and concentrate on your breathing. Let your body sink into the bed. This should feel great after a long day.
- ❑ Breathe in deeply through your nose; let your chest expand and your stomach contract. Feel the energy flowing into your body. As you exhale, press the breath slowly and evenly from your abdomen and chest and out through your nose. Use your stomach muscles, but don't force or strain yourself. Do this for six to eight breaths. Once you have a steady and controlled rhythm, you're ready to begin.
- ❑ Focus your attention on the top of your head and release any pressures there. Slowly move to your forehead, your eyes and your mouth. Free any tension around your jaw, letting your mouth open slightly, if necessary. Maintain an even, deep and controlled breath. Take your time.
- ❑ For each part of your body, do a complete deep inhalation and full exhalation before moving on. Take your time. Try not to rush each breath.
- ❑ Your shoulders and upper back collect a lot of stress during the day, especially if you're working at a computer. Focus on any neck and shoulder strain. Breathe in deeply. As you exhale, slowly release the tension that's collected there.

Continue down your body, concentrating on your arms, abdomen, thighs, calves, lower legs and finally your feet. If you need to, slowly wiggle your fingers and toes to free any tension there. Keep your breathing even, and maintain a steady flow in and out. If you reach any points of particular stress, focus with your breath and release the tension on your exhalation.

The ways and techniques of dealing with insomnia, anxiety, sleep and depression are quite a few. Most people learn to control stress with regular effort. Once the stress levels have come down to the acceptable limits, these problems disappear on their own.

# SECTION 2

# EMOTIONS

*Chapter* **4**

# EMOTIONS

Emotion can also be described as 'Energy-in-Motion'. It is a way of expressing oneself in life. It is essentially the quality of how one relates to life. Emotion is usually considered to be a feeling or reaction to certain important events or thoughts. It is funny that most people who claim to know what an emotion is all about, are sometimes not fully aware of their own emotions. Psychologists have not yet agreed on a definition that applies fully to this strange lot of feelings. Individuals communicate most of their emotions by means of words, a variety of sounds, facial expressions and gestures. For example, anger causes most people to frown, ball their fingers into a fist, and yell.

## Emotions and Fitness

One would ask, and rightly so, what has emotions got to do with fitness. A lot. Emotions are the basis of many reactions and these reactions can trigger off a lot of positive and negative health effects. Have you ever noticed how the adrenaline begins to pump and heart begins to race when you experience anger or fear? Or how wonderful you feel when you are happy? Or how miserable you feel when you are depressed or sad? Emotions are very vital to good health and fitness.

In the early days, scientists tried to discover the link between emotions and health. It was Charles Darwin who developed the theory of natural selection and also studied emotion. Darwin said that emotional behaviour originally served both as an aid to survival and as a method of communicating intentions.

During the 1880's, the American psychologist William James and Danish physiologist Carl G. Lange independently reached another conclusion about emotions. According to their theory, (the *James – Lange theory of emotions)*, people feel emotions only if aware of their own internal physical reactions to events, such as increased heart rate or blood pressure. Though some psychologists believe in this theory, there is little evidence to support it. But the fact remains that a mental well being has a great amount of role to play in the overall development of the body.

## Negative and Positive Emotions

Emotions, as expressed and experienced by humans can be divided into two broad categories. It could be called positive and negative emotions. Now the important thing is **not** judging them as good and bad as the name usually suggests. Positive emotions is all about working on learning more viewpoints, interacting more with others, enjoying making things better. They are emotions, fuelled by an underlying desire for enjoyment and unity. Positive emotions are pleasant, for instance interest, enthusiasm, boredom, love, happiness laughter, empathy, action, curiosity and contentment. Of course there is a range of different emotions in each of those categories.

On the other hand, negative emotions express an attempt or intention to "exclude". Strengthening one's own position at the expense of others, keeping bad stuff away, destroying what is perceived as a threat. Negative emotions are fuelled by an underlying fear of the unknown, a fear of the actions of others, and a need to control them or stop them to avoid being harmed. Negative emotions are, feelings of apathy, grief, fear, hatred, shame, blame, regret, resentment, anger, hostility and loneliness.

It is interesting to note that several American psychologists have devised an independent theory claiming that there are eight basic emotions. These emotions, which can exist at various levels of intensity, are anger, fear, joy, sadness, acceptance, disgust, surprise, and interest or curiosity. They combine to form all other emotions, just as basic colours all others. In our country, we have long known that there are nine kinds of emotions or 'navarasa', so efficiently demonstrated by our bharatnatyam dancers.

Some emotions camouflage as positive or negative, but actually mean the opposite of what is identified. The simple example of this is a type of pity, which appears as genuine concern for others, but in reality might be taking comfort in that somebody else who is in a situation worse than yours. Often what you see as an expressed emotion may not necessarily be the real emotion. It is the underlying mechanism and motivation that counts, more than the superficial outward manifestation.

This might of course lead you to believe that the negative emotions are just something to get rid of. However, it is not that simple. They serve important functions. Basically they show that there is something one doesn't know and can't deal with. If that becomes motivation to then learn it and deal with it that is very useful. If one is always joyful, one might miss noticing things that are wrong. This finally boils down to the fact that though positive and negative emotions are polarities, we can't get rid of one and just keep the other. Ultimately they need to be integrated. One needs to deal with the negative emotions and actually work at transforming them into something more useful and enjoyable.

The aim in processing is to make people more fluid in terms of emotion. Able to use whatever emotion is most appropriate, and being able to use the full range as necessary. Most likely a person who is fluid and flexible will choose to live mostly in a positive frame of mind. But the goal is actually integration, moving beyond the positive/negative idea altogether.

Positive emotions give you energy, while negative emotions deplete your energy. When you are excited and happy and are interacting with people you love and enjoy, you sparkle with energy and enthusiasm, but when you are angry or depressed, or negative for any reason, you feel tired and frustrated, and eventually burned out. This means that, most likely, a person who is fluid and flexible will choose to live mostly in a positive frame of mind. But the goal is actually integration, moving beyond the positive/negative idea altogether.

## Unmasking the Emotions

There is a covert hostility that masks as friendliness, which can often be difficult to assess at first. Likewise, some kinds of anger or tears might look negative, but might really be an expression of involvement and care for the whole.

The negative emotions are useful as motivation for moving away from what one doesn't want. The positive emotions are useful as motivation for moving towards what one does want. Trouble enters when parts of the system get stuck. Particularly when the functions get reversed and the person starts moving towards what she doesn't want. Therefore, stuck negative emotions are a prime target for processing.

People might express all sorts of combinations of these emotions. Some people will be fairly chronically stuck in a negative emotion, like grief for example. Others might be stuck in a positive one, like contentment, and won't be able to experience negative emotions, even when appropriate. Others will in stressful situations react according to certain emotional patterns. Like, a person might have hidden grief or fear that gets triggered by certain circumstances. A casual remark might push a button that unleashes pent-up anger. The aim in processing is to make people more fluid in terms of emotion. Able to use whatever emotion is most appropriate, and being able to use the full range as necessary.

## Positive Emotions Are the Key to Life

Here's the important point. Let's say it takes a thousand units of physical energy to operate your body. If you do not do physical labour, that physical energy can be recycled in your body to produce a hundred units of emotional energy. Emotional energy is a far more refined form of energy, and it is absolutely essential to healthy emotional functioning. If you do not consume all this energy in the expression of negative emotions, such as fear, doubt, anger and resentment, your emotional energies are conserved. If your energy is conserved at one level, your body continues to refine it into higher and better energy. Therefore, your body into 10 units of mental energy will refine a hundred units of emotional energy thus conserved.

You've probably heard someone described as "shaking with anger." When a person is shaking with anger, it is an indication that he or she has burned up the glucose or sugar-based energy in the system, and is actually weak from an angry outburst. Another characteristic of very successful people is that they keep themselves calm much longer than the average person does. They are more relaxed, more genial and more in control of their emotions. They are very aware that expressions of negative emotion deprive them of the energy they need to be effective in the more important things they do. As a result, successful people don't allow themselves to become upset or angry over little things, or even over large things. They remain objective and detached. They stand back and refuse to take things personally. They do not allow themselves to get drawn into arguments or other people's problems. They save their emotional energy for far more productive purposes.

The whole purpose of physical relaxation is to allow yourself to recharge your emotional and mental batteries. You don't engage in physical relaxation so much to relax your physical body; because it's likely you don't work that hard with your body. The aim of rest and relaxation is more to build up your mental and emotional energies and thereby improve the overall quality of your entire life.

Now, here are three things you can do immediately to put these ideas into action.

- ❑ First, keep your thoughts on your dreams and goals, and keep them off the things and people that cause you stress and negative emotions. This is not easy, but it's very important.
- ❑ Second, preserve your emotional energy by staying calm and positive in difficult situations rather than allowing yourself to become upset or angry.
- ❑ Third, take ample time to rest completely so you can recharge your physical and emotional batteries. The better rested you are, the more effective you will be.

## Managing Emotions

The more we learn about the mind-body connection, the more we realize the benefits of having a control over our emotions.

There are three important steps to managing the emotions -

1. **Express gratitude** – Focusing on the positive and practicing thankfulness will crowd out those stressful negative feelings.
2. **Have the courage to cry** – Far from being a sign of weakness, shedding tears is a testimony to your inner strength.
3. **Forgive and forget** – Difficult as you may find it to seek closure; actively forgiving someone — not merely forgetting the transgression — confers countless benefits.

## Expressing gratitude

Seek opportunities to show appreciation for others. Thanks. Such a simple word, and so rarely used - A meaningful gesture that should be employed more often. We are taught, since early childhood, to say "thank you" in response to gifts or kind gestures. Yet, in today's bustling world, we overlook the myriad opportunities to show our appreciation for others and to give back some of what we receive. Say "thanks" to loved ones and people you see every day. This sounds so obvious, but we tend to overlook those closest to us. It's the small things that count.

### *Express appreciation for people you see often and show gratitude to the community*

- Clean up and weed the neighbourhood.
- Volunteer to read to children at your local library.
- Are you a computer whiz? Donate your time to a shelter and help with their computing needs.
- Donate toys, books, games and clothing to the less fortunate.
- Help an elderly lady across the street.

### *Show gratitude to yourself*

Have you ever thought of showing gratitude to yourself? After all, it is your being that is most important. Do something special for yourself, or write in your diary to reinforce your thankful attitude.

Not only does it make others happy, but showing gratitude makes *you* feel great, too. Enjoy the benefits! Be creative! Doing one small kindness for someone else puts a whole new perspective on your day.

## The courage to cry

Despite society's tendency to repress emotion, expressing sadness and grief can be very therapeutic. Not only does grief take courage, but also feeling bad about any situation takes courage in our society of positive thinkers. We are bombarded by so many messages to hide our feelings, unless, of course, they are positive.

### *Embrace your emotions*

A phrase that people often throw around as a way of pushing their feelings aside is: "This is a learning experience." It's true that we learn from all our experiences, no matter how awful. But not everything happens to teach us a lesson. Before we can learn from sad or bad situations, we must first go through them and feel the pain. Denying our feelings only makes recovery longer. The shame or outward denial of feeling bad begins when we are children. When youngsters are angry or depressed, we tell them to stop. Children grow through their emotions and we need to support them and allow that growth.

Tragedies and disappointments are inevitable. When we repress our feelings they come out in other self-destructive ways, including anger, rage, overeating, anorexia, drugs, alcohol, smoking or depression. It takes more courage to feel bad, and let people know how we feel, than to pretend everything is all right. I like to say in public that I feel so much better now that I have the courage to feel bad. If you find yourself feeling down, try a little self-talk: "A (sad, tragic, disappointing, or other appropriate word) thing happened. It is normal to feel bad, and express it. I will be more emotionally healthy and will be able to let go sooner if I feel, rather than deny."

It is also a good idea to talk to a supportive person when you have doubts about the validity of your feelings, a person who will listen and reassure you of your right to feel bad. Make sure the people you ask for support are able to give it. And finally, consider the following questions and how they relate to the experiences of your own life: How will we be able to recognize joy if we have never felt sadness? How can we know fulfilment if we have never known loss? And how can we be human if we never feel?

## What is forgiveness?

Old resentments and failed expectations often interfere with the enjoyment of our lives – try to identify the pain and move on. Forgiveness is letting go of the need for revenge and releasing negative thoughts of bitterness and resentment. If you are a parent, you can provide a wonderful model for your children by forgiving. If they observe your reconciliation with friends or family members who have wronged you, perhaps they will learn not to harbour resentment over the ways in which you may have disappointed them. Even if you are not a parent, forgiveness is still an extremely valuable skill to have.

Forgiveness can be a gift that we give to ourselves. Here are some easy steps towards forgiveness:

- Acknowledge your own inner pain.
- Express your emotions in non-hurtful ways without yelling or attacking.
- Protect yourself from further victimization.
- Try to understand the point of view and motivations of the person to be forgiven; replace anger with compassion.
- Forgive yourself for your role in a difficult relationship, and then decide whether or not to remain in the relationship.

Perform the overt act of forgiveness verbally or in writing. If the person you want to forgive is dead or unreachable, you can still write down your feelings in letter form.

## Expressing Negative Emotions

Just as a termite eats silently into the core of wood, reducing it to worthless powder, negative emotions reduce the human soul into worthless element. They eat into the psyche, ravaging the health and happiness of the person. Why should one want to cling on to negative emotions like anger, frustration, fear or disgust?

At the same time, there is no need for anyone to feel ashamed about the negative emotions that arise in the mind, from time to time. We neither are super humans nor saints. We are normal human beings who are likely to suffer from various kinds of emotions, some good some bad. The trick is not to succumb to the negative emotions but gain control over them. To do so, one must understand the power of positive thinking and positive emotions. An unhappy person sees only misery all around him while a happy person detects happiness all around.

Negativity or negative emotions do nothing but harm to the mind and body. Agreed that it is not an easy task to control one's emotions but it is a process that can bring joy in our lives, forever.

## Expressing Anger

Anger is one of the most destructive of all emotions. It raises blood pressure, disturbs mental equilibrium and plays havoc with general health. An angry person cannot make rational decisions. Choleric people are prone to ulcers, hypertension, backache, migraine and heart problems. Suppressing anger is detrimental to overall well being. It can lead to bowel problems, respiratory ills and skin flare–ups. Expressing anger and ventilating angry feelings is the first step towards control of that emotion. Women are much more likely than men to turn anger inwards and blame themselves, thus becoming depressed. There are many ways by which one can get rid of anger without hurting anyone.

Anger comes in many shapes and forms. For instance –

- Annoyance
- Disappointment.
- Hurt.
- Frustration.
- Harassment.
- Threats.
- Tragedy

## Keep-cool Tips

Here are some ways to come to terms with anger and deal with it without losing your temper:

- Ignore anger provokers.
- Talk quietly and breathe deeply.
- Count ten before you react.
- State what is making you angry, then stop talking.
- A drink of cold water will literally help you cool off.
- Work your anger out on punching bags like soft cushions and pillows. Working it out at the gym or at the playfield is also a very good idea.
- Learn to analyse what it is that makes you angry and why. Recognising the triggers can help keep anger under control.

## Channelling Emotions

Perhaps one of the most interesting words today, is emotion. It is categorised, celebrated, vilified, repressed, manipulated, humiliated, adored, and ignored. Rarely, if ever, are they honoured. As a matter of fact it also happens to be the least understood and over analysed aspects of human life.

There are lots of theories, each adding their own aspect to the word. Many teachings split emotions into categories like good and bad and then spend enormous amounts of time and energy in convincing people to agree with them.

The only problem is that the therapies and teachings can't seem to agree on which emotions are right, and which are wrong. Some religions and teachings shun all emotions, while others shun only anger and fear. Most New Age teachings make do with one emotion (joy), and strive to sublimate the rest. In our society, the "bad" emotion is grief. After a few hundred years of repression, we have become a cold-hearted people, mesmerized by, but incapable of accepting, death.

Expressing the emotions is better than repressing them, because it allows a flow of truthfulness in the body and spirit. If emotions are very strong, however, expressing them can create both exterior and interior turmoil. The exterior turmoil occurs when we pour our strong emotions all over some unfortunate soul and try to make him or her responsible for our mood. The interior turmoil occurs when we realize we have startled or hurt someone with our outpouring, which makes us feel dismayed and ashamed of ourselves. Then we either repress the emotions again, or express them even more loudly, neither of which will help anyone.

Often, our strong emotions make us lash out and blame others for our feelings, ("You made me angry, you made me cry!"). Expressing strong emotions can be damaging to our egos. So, what's left? If we can't repress emotions without getting into trouble, and we can't express them either, what can we do, live in a cave? No. We can channel our emotions.

When we express our emotions, we hand them over to the outside world, where we hope they will be noticed, honoured, healed, and transformed into something bright and beautiful. Emotional expression relies on the exterior world and on other people to translate and alter emotional messages into action. When we repress emotions, we hand them over to the interior world, where we hope they will be taken care of, healed, and transformed into something more acceptable to us. Emotional repression relies on the unconscious, interior world to accept and do something with the emotion.

Neither hand-off works for very long. Emotional expression makes us unworkably dependent on therapists, books, friends, family members, clergy, and external action for emotional relief and release. Since all of these exterior people or supports can leave or be taken away, we emotion-expressers can become stuck with a life full of feelings, but no emotional skills of our own, and nowhere to go with the feelings and energies we have.

Emotional repression, on the other hand, makes us unworkably dependent on a body or an unconscious that can only hold so much repressed material before it has to get rid of something. When you hand off your emotional responsibilities to your body, it stores them somewhere until they eventually show up as pain or illness. If you hand- off to your unconscious and tell it, "No anger or grief, okay?" your unconscious works very hard to obey you, but it has to create something else with all your angry, grieving energy. Suicidal urges usually do the trick.

Both the expression and repression of emotion have serious drawbacks. The hand-off never works. On the other hand, when you listen to, honour, and channel your emotions, you don't need to hand them off to anyone or anything. Emotional channelling lets you handle your emotions yourself. When you are able to take care of your own emotions, they will take care of you in ways you may not be able to believe right now.

All emotions are messages from our unconscious aspects to our conscious ones. Emotions may spring from our bodies, from our deep memories, or from unused and unnoticed aspects of our psyches. Strong or uncontrollable emotions carry, not just truth, but enormous amounts of energy. Strong emotions contribute the energy we need to heal ourselves and evolve. Strong emotions are the energetic warehouse of the soul.

All emotions are tools for our use, if we accept them, channel them responsibly, and take the time to listen to their healing messages. Not surprisingly, the "bad" emotions can bring us amazing insights, because they carry so much energy with them. Anger and fury can signal a lack of boundaries, and then contribute the energy to rebuild those boundaries into strong protectors. Sadness and despair can signal an arid harshness in the self or the environment, and then contribute the healing fluidity that was missing. Anxiety, fear, and terror can signal the presence of dangerously wrong people, ideas, or environments, and then contribute protection, or the energy to move out of harm's way.

Emotional channelling reminds us that a healthy psyche is a complete one. Completeness includes light and dark, good and bad, love and hate, perfection and flaws, solemnity and silliness, wisdom and idiocy, and everything else. If you ignore your own shadowy emotions and try to hide them, or throw them out with the trash, they may loom up and attack you with your own repressed energy. Emotional channelling does not interfere with the expression of our needs, feelings, and moods to the aware and supportive people in our lives. Rather, it offers a stronger (and more personally empowering) support. When we work with the energetic material of our own emotions, we no longer need to rely on others to help us deal with or validate them.

In order to remain whole and alive from this moment forward, you'll need an environment that lets you cry when you're sad, squeal and jump when you're exhilarated, move quickly when you're anxious, protect yourself when you're fearful, stomp and snap when you're angry, dance when you're happy, and grieve when you lose someone or something. Whole people accept and honour all human emotions.

Your life right now may not be whole, but when you commit to channelling your emotions, you will move toward completeness. Your inner life, at least, will be the environment where you will be free to feel.

*Chapter* **5**

# RELAXATION TECHNIQUES

## BREATH CONTROL

Stress and relaxation are two sides of the same coin and both are necessary for a healthy life. When they are in balance all is well, but if stress predominates, illness often develops – the possible consequences can range from headaches, anxiety and lethargy to heart attacks, ulcers or cancer. While experts agree that stress plays a part in the onset of many disorders, it is also an accepted truth that not all stress is bad. Even events like getting married, receiving a promotion, having a baby are stressful, but good for you. All stress comes from two basic sources: physical activity and mental or emotional activity.

### Stress Management Techniques

Stress management can be done through Mental and physical techniques. Mental techniques includes various methods like meditation, Pranayam, imagery, self hypnosis, Reiki, Vipassana etc. while physical methods are mainly to do with physical exercises of various kinds e.g. aerobics, Tai chi etc.

### Choosing a Technique

To many people, relaxation does not come naturally, though stress does. Because of this, most people have to make a special effort to learn how to relax. Each individual must choose from the combination of the techniques that are available, until you find those that suit you and your lifestyle; when you try any particular one, concentrate on what you personally want out of it, and remember that you are more likely to succeed if you choose a method and stick to it.

Some of the techniques described have primarily a mental effect; others mainly affect the body. Many of the mental techniques originate in the East, where they have been used for centuries to achieve deep relaxation, inner peace and tranquillity. If you feel that such qualities are missing in your life try one of these techniques – meditation, for example.

Other techniques are based on achieving a physical harmony and balance that will, in turn, affect mental well-being. If you find it easier to achieve physical and mental relaxation through movement or 'doing something', these are the techniques for you.

Whichever techniques you choose, persevere with them for a while before trying another one, quick changes are in themselves a sign of stress.

## Breathing Techniques

The importance of correct breathing has been recognised since beginning of history. The Shaman, the wise men and witch doctors of ancient times used breathing techniques to induce trances or to improve performance and correct breathing was and still is considered to be vital for good health, in eastern medicine. It is also thought to be essential if one is to progress to the higher levels of skills in meditational and martial arts and in the achievement of the 'asanas' or postures taken up during T'ai Chi and yoga exercise, for example. Today, it is generally recognised that correct breathing has an important role to play, in particular, in helping to reduce levels of stress as well as its signs and symptoms.

The environmental strains of modern urban life have made breathing techniques even more important than they have been in the past since the air that we take into our bodies is polluted with smoke and chemicals that can damage lung tissues. Polluted air is dangerously low in oxygen, vital for the physical and the mental health of the body – and low in the atmospheric ions that are linked with positive health.

Since it is impractical for the majority of us to start a new life in the less polluted countryside, it is vitally important that we breathe as efficiently as possible. During inspiration (breathing in), air is drawn into the lungs, where it fills tiny air sacs that are surrounded by a network of miniscule blood vessels. The blood then absorbs the oxygen and transports it around the body to supply every cell. As the oxygen is absorbed, the blood passes carbon di-oxide- the waste product of energy released from the cells-back into the air, to be removed from the body during expiration (breathing out).

If the process is less than efficient, blood oxygen levels become low, and blood carbon-di-oxide levels become high. Too little oxygen and too much carbon-di-oxide and the cells will die, those of the brain and nervous system being particularly vulnerable.

Though we all breathe by instinct, most people use only about half their lung capacity, the result being that the air sacs (alveoli) absorb too little oxygen, leaving an excess of carbon di oxide in the tissues which is reabsorbed by the blood. Conversely, panic or anxiety attacks, when breathing can become so shallow and rapid; a condition known as hyperventilation – that the body expels too much carbon di oxide, are a problem for some people. With practice, though, breathing can be made more efficient, so that hyperventilation during anxiety can be avoided by breathing control, thereby reducing stress and leading to general well being.

## Importance of Breathing

Breathing is important for two reasons. It is the only means to supply our bodies and its various organs with the supply of oxygen, which is vital for our survival. The second function of breathing is that it is one means to get rid of waste products and toxins from the body.

## Why is Oxygen Vital

Oxygen is the most vital nutrient for our bodies. It is essential for the integrity of the brain, nerves, glands and internal organs. We can do without food for weeks and without water for days, but without oxygen, we will die within a few minutes. If the brain does not get proper supply of this essential nutrient, it will result in the degradation of all vital organs in the body.

The brain requires more oxygen than any other organ. If it doesn't get enough, the result is mental sluggishness, negative thoughts and depression and, eventually, vision and hearing decline.

Yogis realized the vital importance of an adequate oxygen supply thousands of years ago. They developed and perfected various breathing techniques. These breathing exercises are particularly important for people who have sedentary jobs and spend most of the day in offices. Their brains are oxygen starved and their bodies are just 'getting by'. They feel tired, nervous and irritable and are not very productive. On top of that, they sleep badly at night, so they get a bad start to the next day, continuing the cycle. This situation also lowers their immune system, making them susceptible to catching colds, flu and other infections.

## Oxygen Purifies the Blood Stream

One of the major secrets of vitality and rejuvenation is a purified blood stream. The quickest and most effective way to purify the blood stream is by taking in extra supplies of oxygen from the air we breathe. The breathing exercises described in here are the most effective methods ever devised for saturating the blood with extra oxygen. Oxygen bums up the waste products (toxins) in the body, as well as recharging the body's batteries (the solar plexus). In fact, most of our energy requirements come not from food but from the air we breathe. By purifying the blood stream, every part of the body benefits, as well as the mind. Your complexion will become clearer and brighter and wrinkles will begin to fade away. In short, rejuvenation will start to occur.

Scientists have known for a long time that there exists a strong connection between respiration and mental states. Improper breathing produces diminished mental ability. It is known that mental tensions produce restricted breathing. A normally sedentary person, when confronted with a perplexing problem, tends to lean forward, draw his arms together, and bend his head down. All these body postures results in reduced lung capacity.

We become fatigued from the decreased circulation of the blood and from the decreased availability of oxygen for the blood because we have almost stopped breathing. As our duties, responsibilities and their attendant problems become more demanding, we develop habits of forgetting to breathe.

## What's Wrong With The Way We Breath?

Our breathing is too shallow and too quick. We are not taking in sufficient oxygen and we are not eliminating sufficient carbon dioxide. , As a result, our bodies are oxygen starved, and a toxic build-up occurs.

Shallow breathing does not exercise the lungs enough, so they lose some of their function, causing a further reduction in vitality. Animals, which breathe slowly, live the longest; the elephant is a good example.

We need to breathe more slowly and deeply. Quick shallow breathing results in oxygen starvation which leads to reduced vitality, premature ageing, poor immune system and a myriad of other factors. Shallow breathing also results in reduced vitality, since oxygen is essential for the production of energy in the body, and increased disease. Our resistance to disease is reduced, since oxygen is essential for healthy cells. This means we catch more colds and develop other ailments more easily. Lack of sufficient oxygen to the cells is a major contributing factor in cancer, heart disease and strokes.

### Basic method

Start by learning correct breathing techniques when lying down, alone and without distractions. Once you have mastered the technique, it can be practiced in any position, anywhere – eventually it will become a habit.

1. Put on loose, comfortable clothes and lie on your back on the floor, using a mat if more comfortable, or on your bed.
2. Place both your hands on the lower edges of your ribs, with fingers nearly touching.

3. Relax your body.
4. Breathe in deeply and smoothly through your nostrils. Feel your diaphragm pulling out and down, your stomach rising and your ribs expanding upwards and outwards. Hold the breath for a few seconds.
5. Breathe out smoothly. This requires no muscular activity, since all that happens is that the diaphragm and the muscles of the chest let go, but try to ensure that all the air that you inhaled is expelled. The ribs collapse down and in; the stomach lowers.
6. Repeat three or four times, then relax and breathe naturally for a few minutes, before starting the sequence once again.

Note:
- ❒ Your shoulders should remain stationary during breathing. Many people, especially women breathe solely into their upper lobes by raising and lowering their shoulders. This does not give the body an adequate supply of oxygen and is a common symptom of stress.
- ❒ If you feel heady and faint during the breathing exercises, relax and breathe naturally for a few minutes – the sensation passes quickly and is the result of the brain receiving an unusually large amount of oxygen.

## Breathing while sitting

1. Make sure you are sitting comfortably with your spine straight.
2. Relax your shoulders and place your hands loosely on your lap.
3. Breathe using the same basic method as for lying down.
4. Feel the air filling your lungs, right down to the bottom lobes.
5. Check your shoulders – they should not be moving up and down.
6. If you feel that you are not filling your lungs fully, place your hands on the bottom edge of the ribs, and over the stomach and check that your ribs and stomach are expanding fully under your fingers as you breathe

in. breathe like this a few times until you sense the movement and then return your hands to your lap.

## Breathing while walking

1. Walk at a steady pace, letting your hands swing loosely by your side.
2. Breathe in deeply – as in the basic method- for a certain number of paces, hold the breath for half that number and breathe out gradually for the same number. Find which number of paces feels right for you.
3. Maintain the rhythm and repeat the exercise five times. Then relax and breathe naturally.
4. Repeat the whole exercise a few times during each walk.

## Healing breath

This method of healing in used in all branches of eastern medicine, though not in orthodox western medicine. It involves breathing in the *chi,* as Chinese and Japanese medicine calls the 'life force', or the *prana,* as Indian medicine names it, into the lungs and visualising it flowing from them first into the solar plexus and then to the area to be healed. During exhalation the disease is visualised flowing out of the body.

## Re-energising breath

These two exercises in breathing will first perform a releasing function on your body and mind and then re-charge them. The second exercise is especially structured to boost your vitality but it should be used sparingly to prevent hyperventilation.

- ❑ Breathe in deeply through an open mouth and sigh out with a relaxed throat. Your upper back widens on the inhale and releases on the exhale. Don't worry if you yawn; it's your body's homeostatic mechanism correcting your oxygen and carbon dioxide balance.
- ❑ Open your mouth wide, inhale deeply and let the air out in a big 'hah'. Repeat a few times quickly. If you feel light-headed, breathe normally through your nose. Tingling in your mouth or fingers is a normal reaction to shifting levels of oxygen and carbon dioxide.

## A tension-relaxer

This exercise is particularly useful, since it only takes a few minutes and can be performed anywhere, at any time.

1. Stand up with your hands hanging loosely by your side.
2. Breathe in slowly through your nostrils, tensing all your muscles at the same time.
3. Hunch your shoulders up to your ears, clench your hands as hard as possible, tighten your stomach muscles, clench your buttocks and raise yourself up on to tiptoe.
4. Hold this position to the count of five. Fix your eye on something straight ahead to help you balance.
5. Slowly breathe out through your nostrils and at the same time relax all your muscles, so that by the time you have fully exhaled your shoulders are down, your hands are floppy, your stomach is relaxed and your knees are slightly bent.
6. Repeat five times.

## Alternate nose breathing

This breathing technique is recommended for calming the spirit and the mind. The sun and moon are seen here as symbols of the positive and negative, and this technique shows you how to inhale the positive energy of the sun and exhale the negative waste products of the body.

1. Sit in an upright position –cross-legged if you can manage it, otherwise sit on a firm backed chair.
2. Pinch your nostrils shut with your right hand, the thumb closing the right nostril and the index and middle finger closing the left nostril. Only gentle pressure is needed, so do not pinch too hard.
3. Breathe through your mouth as you practise opening and closing the nostrils alternately.
4. When you have learnt how to do this, inhale deeply and slowly as for the basic method through your right nostril – keep the left nostril firmly closed.
5. Hold for the amount of time it took you to inhale – tough not if it feels uncomfortable.

6. Exhale gradually through your left nostril again for the same length of time it took to inhale. The comparative ratio for these three motions – breathing in, holding, then breathing out – is therefore 1:1:1. This rhythm can take a while to master, but the control it engenders and the results are worthwhile. Traditionally, those advanced in yoga use a ratio of 1:4:2, but without specialised training you should not try to go beyond 1:2:2.
7. Breathe in this way five times and then use the left nostril to inhale and the right nostril to exhale and repeat.
8. Breathe twice through both nostrils deeply and fully.
9. Relax totally in the same position and feel the tension disappearing.

## De-stressing breath

The more stressed out we are, the tighter we hold ourselves, especially in the jaw, chest and diaphragm. If we breathe deeply, the oxygen flows, and we can think and feel more clearly.

This exercise will help you de-stress and unwind.

- ❑ Sit cross-legged on the floor, or in a chair with your feet flat on the ground, head straight and chin parallel to the floor.
- ❑ Inhale slowly through your nose, filling your abdomen, ribs and chest. Then blow out steadily though puckered lips until your lungs are empty.
- ❑ Breathe in again, feeling your torso muscles move like a bellows. Imagine expelling tension from your body.

## Pranayama: The Breathing Exercises of Yoga

Pranayama, as traditionally conceived, involves much more than merely breathing for relaxation. Pranayama is a term with a wide range of meanings. Patanjali defines pranayama as "the regulation of the incoming and outgoing flow of breath with retention." It is to be practised only after perfection in asana is attained. Pranayama also denotes cosmic power, or the power of the entire universe, which manifests itself as conscious living being in us through the phenomenon of breathing.

The word pranayama consists of two parts: prana and ayama. **Ayama** means stretch, extension, expansion, length, breadth, regulation, prolongation, restraint and control and describes the action of pranayama. **Prana** is energy, when the self-energizing force embraces the body. When this self-energizing force embraces the body with extension, expansion and control, it is pranayama.

**Prana** - Prana is an auto-energizing force, which creates a magnetic field in the form of the Universe and plays with it, both to maintain, and to destroy for further creation. It acts as physical energy, mental energy, where the mind gathers information; and as intellectual energy, where information is examined and filtered. Prana also acts as sexual energy, spiritual energy and cosmic energy. All that vibrates in this Universe is prana: heat, light, gravity, magnetism, vigour, power, vitality, electricity, life and spirit are all forms of prana. It is the cosmic personality, potent in all beings and non-beings. It is the prime mover of all activity. It is the wealth of life.

## AUTOGENIC RELAXATION TECHNIQUES

### Autogenic Relaxation

Autogenics, as the name suggests, are self-generated suggestions your mind gives your body to relax. It is a quick and portable relaxation technique that pin-points body regions that need to relax. For example: shoulders, jaw, or neck muscles may be the first area of your body to tense when you are stressed. Autogenic relaxation of any one of these areas could be done with just a minute or two of concentrated relaxation. Here is how this works.

### Autogenics Script

- Sit is a comfortable chair and close your eyes. Begin by taking a few deep breaths. In your mind's eye, pin-point the area of your body you would like to relax. See the tension this area is currently holding: tight muscles, restricted blood flow or contractions. Now, in your mind's eye, see this same area of your body opening or calming.

- ❑ Repeat the sentence below for 6 or more times. Repeat each command until the desired result is felt and then continue to the next one. "My legs and arms are heavy". "My legs and arms are warm". "My heart is steady and calm". "My breathing is regular and calm." "My forehead is cool and clear."

It may take quite a few sessions to achieve the correct state of relaxation but it is worth persevering, since this is such a simple technique that can be practiced anywhere, and it will leave you feeling calm and capable.

## STATIC RELAXATION TECHNIQUES

### Exercise Regularly

Taking frequent effective exercise is probably one of the best physical stress-reduction techniques available. Exercise not only improves your health and reduces stress it also relaxes tense muscles and helps you to sleep.

Exercise has a number of other positive benefits:

- ❑ It improves blood flow to your brain, bringing additional sugars and oxygen which may be needed when you are thinking intensely.
- ❑ When you think hard, the neurones of your brain function more intensely. As they do this they build up toxic waste products that cause foggy thinking in the short term, and can damage the brain in the long term. By exercising you speed the flow of blood through your brain, moving these waste products faster. You also improve this blood flow so that even when you are not exercising, waste is eliminated more efficiently.
- ❑ It can cause release of chemicals called endorphins into your blood stream. These give you a feeling of happiness and well-being.

Studies indicate that many traditionally recommended forms of exercise actually damage your body over the medium or long term. It is worth finding reputable and up-to-date sources of advice on exercise, possibly from your doctor, and then having a customised exercise plan drawn up for you.

An important thing to remember is that exercise should be fun - if you do not enjoy it, then you will probably not keep doing it.

## Basic Technique

A self-help technique to reduce accumulated stress in the body, by progressively contracting and relaxing the muscle groups that store tension. While it is essential that our muscles maintain a certain amount of tension to support posture and movement, it is when our bodies have to move unnaturally or under stress that the result can be extra, unnecessary tension in certain muscles – for example, in neck and shoulders. This itself causes symptoms of stress headaches, aches and pains and general tiredness, for example- and so the vicious circle is established.

To break out of this circle we need to know how to release excess tension from the muscles – this is the first step in relaxation, and is used in all the various techniques. To succeed, however, one important lesson should be borne in mind; that is, a recognition that most of the time we tend to concentrate on what is happening in the outside world around us, whereas the essence of relaxation is to bring that focus back inside ourselves, so that we may become sensitive to the tensions within and begin to relieve them.

## Method

Put on loose, comfortable clothes, making sure that your feet are warm.

1. Lie down in a quiet, warm, dark room, using the floor, a mat or a firm bed – this is perhaps the best position for a beginner, though alternative positions are given below. Place a pillow or cushion under your head and knees. Either let your hands and arms rest by your side or gently upon your stomach, whichever feels the most comfortable.
2. Check that you feel really comfortable. If necessary, use more pillows – perhaps under your feet and forearms.

Only start the technique once you are certain of your comfort.

3. Relax and let your mind go blank. Take a couple of deep breaths and sigh the air away.
4. Now you are ready to start reducing tension in your muscles. The technique involves letting go of all the muscles in the body, starting at the toes, working gradually up the body and ending with the face. To begin, concentrate on your left foot. Tense all the muscles – curling the toes and scrunching the foot. Hold for a few seconds. Let go, and make them feel floppy, heavy and warm, as if they are sinking in to the pillow. It may take a little practice to perfect this technique, but it will come if you persevere.
5. Move onto the calf muscles on the left leg. Tense the muscles, hold and let go. Feel the heaviness and warmth of the leg and foot.
6. Apply the same technique on the left thigh. Concentrate on the left leg – does it feel heavy, warm, and relaxed. Is it sinking into the floor or bed? If the answers are 'no', tense the whole leg, hold it in tension until it feels difficult to hold the position any longer, then let go completely.
7. Repeat the same process with the right leg.
8. When both legs feel heavy and numb, continue moving up the body. Clench your buttocks tightly and let go; pull in your stomach muscles, hold tight, relax; let them fallback towards the spine into the floor or bed. Feel the warmth spreading up your body.
9. Breathe deeply and evenly a few times, then sigh the breath away; imagine you are sighing all the tension out of your body.
10. Move on to your left hand, squeeze your hand into a fist, hold tight and let go. Tighten the muscles in the arm, let them flop. Continue with your right arm. Repeat if the arms are not relaxed and heavy. They should feel numb and impossible to move.

11. Hunch your shoulders up towards your ears, hold, let go; let them sink into the floor. It may be necessary to repeat this movement a few times as we hold a lot of tension in our shoulders. Pull the shoulders up towards the ceiling and let them flop back into the ground. Repeat a couple of times.
12. Rock your head gently from side to side in order to loosen the neck. Feel the total relaxation of the body, breathe deeply a few times. Relax, feel the warmth and quiet,
13. The face is the most difficult part of the body to relax; yawn widely with an open mouth, let go; purse the lips out in a pout, then relax; frown fiercely, let go; move the scalp by raising the eyebrows, then relax.
14. The whole body should now be relaxed. Breathe evenly in and out, saying to yourself with each breath that you feel more and more relaxed, peaceful and warm.
15. Rest, relaxed and warm for around 15 minutes. Do not jump up and start racing around. Slowly and gently, stretch and give yourself a shake before allowing the outside world to impinge on your mind

## Relaxation Checklist

Once you have mastered the basic relaxation techniques, you can apply them almost anywhere. It is important, though, to cultivate an awareness of how your body feels throughout the day, so that you can learn to recognise the difference between normal and unnatural amounts of tension. Once you begin to notice when and where you tense up, you can pinpoint your exercises to relax those muscle groups that are affected.

1. Don't leap out of bed in the morning late, with too much to do before you start the day. Set the alarm just 5 minute earlier to give yourself time to relax.
2. Plan to have time to yourself at home – when the children are at school, for example, or playing peacefully. Let the family know that certain times of

the day are 'your time' – then lie down or sink into a chair and empty your mind of all household and work problems. Concentrate on how your body feels and note areas of tension; then use the relaxation technique.

3. Watch out for tension in your shoulders and arms when driving a car. Are you gripping the steering wheel, sitting bolt upright and frowning? At traffic lights or in a traffic jam, take a few seconds to concentrate on yourself; hunch the shoulders up, then let them flop down; slacken your grip on the steering wheel; relax back into your seat and feel the tension leave your body. Breathe slowly and deeply – it is difficult to become angry and frustrated while you are doing this.

## DYNAMIC RELAXATION TECHNIQUES

### Stretching

One of the quickest responses our body has to stress is increased muscle tension and contraction. The physiologic reason for this muscular activity is to prepare us for fight or flight but, in reality, few of our modern day stresses are resolved by either. When muscle tension continues for long periods without physical release a low, or even moderate, level of chronic pain may develop, especially in the shoulders, neck and lower back. To break the contraction cycle and relax these muscle areas, stretch them each 3 or more times each week.

### Neck Stretch

Drop your head to extend your right ear toward your right shoulder. Hold this position 10 to 20 seconds. From this position, roll your head forward to touch your chin to your chest. Hold this position 10 to 20 seconds. From this position, roll your head to the left to extend your left ear toward your left shoulder. Hold this position 10 to 20 seconds. From this position, roll your head forward again to touch your chin to your chest. Hold this position 10 to 20 seconds. From this position, lift your head to centre on top of your shoulders.

## Upper Back Stretch

Stand in open doorway. Grab onto the backside of the doorframe with both your right and left hands. Holding on securely, lean forward until you feel the stretch across your chest. Hold the stretch 20 to 30 seconds.

## Lower Back Stretch

Lie down on a firm surface onto your back. Keep one leg straight for support. Bend the other knee and place both hands behind it. (Do not place hands over the kneecap. Clasp hands behind the knee.) Gently pull the bent knee up toward your chest, letting its lower leg relax. Relax your head back onto the floor. Hold this stretch with firm, consistent pressure by the supporting hands for 20 to 30 seconds. The muscles in your lower back should feel a stretch but no pain. If you feel pain, reduce the amount of stretch until you are comfortable again. Repeat this stretch on the other side.

## Visualization

Like autogenics, visualization uses the power of your mind's eye and inner voice to bring about relaxation. Visualization is the imagery of any location that, to you, is peaceful and stress-free. Your peaceful image can be brought to your consciousness at anytime (in a traffic jam, a tense time at the office) for a quick moment of tension release. Advance practice will allow you to call upon this imagery more effectively at times of stress. For its deepest effect, visualization is done in combination with progressive relaxation. Once deeply relaxed, spend a few minutes imagining the peaceful location you wish to "visit". The more detail you add to your image, the more real it will seem to your mind.

## Positive Thinking

Stress can be triggered by our own negative thoughts just as easily as by outside events. Our body doesn't distinguish between real and imagined threats. If we tell ourself we are going to have trouble with something and that it won't turn out well, we become tense, anxious and prepare for the worse.

On the other hand, if we visualize a good outcome, even if it requires some hard work to achieve, our stress level will be lower in approaching the task. Affirmations are powerful to help redirect thoughts, which are headed on a downward course. They are an important tool for effective stress management.

## Relaxation Tips:

- ❑ **Laughter and smile** – Laughter releases tension, eases difficult situations, relieves embarrassment, and diffuses temper. It lightens up your face and dissolves the lines caused by frowns and tension, making you more attractive to others in an instant; it is extremely difficult for someone to feel annoyed when faced with a smile. Laughter renews hope and helps you to view problems in a more positive and objective manner.
- ❑ **Stop worrying** – either about real or imagined problems. Worrying never achieves anything but heartache, lines on your face and sleepless nights. This is easier said than done, true, but try practising certain tricks to prevent your mind from dwelling on any one problem; watch a comedy; play a complicated game of patience; cook a new and difficult dish; or read a challenging book.
- ❑ **Take pleasure in little things** – look out for simple, everyday occurrences and relish them: a smile on a child's face, a funny hairstyle; a chance meeting; an unexpected compliment, a joke; a beautiful sunset.
- ❑ **Stimulate your mind** – if you have repetitive and boring job, try to change your job to one that suits your personality, because an unsatisfactory and undemanding job can cause a considerable amount of stress. In the mean time take up an exciting hobby, join a club or take a course.
- ❑ **Pamper yourself** – do not wait for others to suggest that you do so, because you might wait too long, and you know what you like and need. Insist on your own chosen method; it might be a hot bath, a brisk walk in the rain, a good book or an evening chat with a friend.

- ❑ **Walk tall** - doing so will almost definitely fool others, and may eventually fool you. Also, it is more difficult to feel depressed and unsure of yourself if you are holding your head high to face the world.
- ❑ **Be realistic** - it is no good trying to alter your basic personality; learn to manage it, and to utilize its strengths and accept its weaknesses.
- ❑ **Live in the present** - we should learn from our past mistakes but should not carry them around with us. Holding on to past errors is as futile as refusing to let go of an unwieldy suitcase full of outgrown clothes.
- ❑ **Learn to say 'no'** - both at work and at home, to the children, to your partner and to your boss. You are no good to anyone when you are exhausted, resentful and over-stretched. People will respect you more if you are straightforward and decisive.
- ❑ **Exercise** - any form of exercise is useful for reducing any sudden increase in tension or stress and setting the body back on to an even keel. Go for a walk, take a swim, dance, play tennis or scrub the kitchen floor.
- ❑ **Prioritise** - at home, at work and in social situations, try to strike a balance between the imperatives of these three basic aspects of a healthy life. In each area, pay attention to the important things first, because the stress of 'unfinished business' is usually worse than solving the problem. Avoid using trivialities to put off confronting important issues.
- ❑ **Plan ahead for your retirement** - join local organizations, for example, or take up part time voluntary work. Once retired, plan your day, not forgetting time for yourself, until the change from organised work to voluntary discipline has become a habit.
- ❑ **Seeking professional help** - we all have different stress levels. It is not a sign of weakness to suffer from stress, but more often a sign of overwhelming willpower and determination not to give in or stubbornness in admitting that one is not perfect or invincible.

*Chapter* **6**

# REIKI

Reiki is a Japanese form of healing that is becoming increasingly popular worldwide. What makes Reiki unique is that it incorporates elements of just about every other alternative healing practices such as spiritual healing, auras, crystals, chakra balancing, meditation, aromatherapy, naturopathy, and homeopathy.

Reiki involves the transfer of energy from practitioner to patient to enhance the body's natural ability to heal itself through the balancing of energy. Reiki utilizes specific techniques for restoring and balancing the natural life force energy within the body. It is a holistic, natural, hands-on energy healing system that touches on all levels: body, mind, and spirit. Reiki (pronounced ray-key) is a Japanese word representing universal life energy, the energy that is all around us. It is derived from rei, meaning "free passage" or "transcendental spirit" and ki, meaning "vital life force energy" or " universal life energy".

## What is Reiki

Reiki practitioners channel energy in a particular pattern to heal and harmonize. Unlike other healing therapies based on the premise of a human energy field, reiki seeks to restore order to the body whose vital energy has become unbalanced.

Reiki energy has several basic effects: it brings about deep relaxation, destroys energy blockages, detoxifies the system, provides new vitality in the form of healing universal life energy, and increases the vibrational frequency of the body.

The laying of hands is used in Reiki therapy also as in spiritual healing. There is a difference though. In spiritual healing, a person with a strong energy field places the hands above a particular part of the recipient's body in order to release energy into it. So, here the healer is the one who is sending out the energy. In Reiki, however, the healer places the hands above the part; however, it is the recipient that draws the energy as needed. Thus, in this case, the individual takes an active part as opposed to a passive part in spiritual healing. The individual takes responsibility for his or her healing. The recipient identifies the needs and caters to them by drawing energy as needed. Although there are a few positions in which the practitioner is in contact with the patient (such as cradling the head), most reiki treatments do not involve actual touching. The practitioner holds his or her hands a few inches or farther away from the patient's body and manipulates the energy field from there.

## History of Reiki

Reiki is believed to have begun in Tibet several thousand years ago. Seers in the Orient studied energies and developed a system of sounds and symbols for universal healing energies. Various healing systems, which crossed many different cultures, emerged from this single root system. Unfortunately, the original source itself was forgotten.

Dr. Mikao Usui, a Japanese Christian educator in Kyoto, Japan, rediscovered the root system in the mid- to late 1800s. He began an extensive twenty-one-year study of the healing phenomena of history's greatest spiritual leaders. He also studied ancient sutras (Buddhist teachings written in Sanskrit). He discovered ancient sounds and symbols that are linked directly to the human body and nervous system, which activate the universal life energy for healing. Usui then underwent a metaphysical experience and became empowered to use these sounds and symbols to heal. He called this form of healing Reiki and taught it throughout Japan until his death around 1893.

## Benefits of Reiki

The whole body reiki is used to treat the whole body to achieve the relaxation and with it the removal of blockages in energy flow and the dispersal of toxins.

Long-term whole-body reiki will restore the general condition of the body. The energy channels are opened to allow the body to deal properly and naturally with both stress and the build-up of toxins. It will help you to cope with anxiety and depression. Reiki has been known to provide its practitioners with the ability to deal with stressful situations. You will gain a positive outlook on life. Once the blockages and toxins have been removed from the system, the scope for personal advancement and growth becomes available. In general, the better metabolic functioning afforded by reiki therapy means that benefits and improvements may be experienced in many ways.

## Meditation with Reiki

Reiki is said to assist in the concentration required for meditation, with the flow of energy aiding relaxation. There are some positions that can be adopted in reiki meditation to achieve particular goals. In the first position the legs are drawn up and the soles of the feet put together with the knees falling apart. This can be done while lying down or sitting against a wall or chair. The hands adopt a praying gesture. This is meant to complete the circuit of energy, allowing a flow around the body. The reiki energy removes any blockages and performed regularly, this becomes a powerful meditation exercise. It can be done for short periods initially, just a couple of minutes, and then built up in small increases. Group meditation is also possible with reiki, in which the participants stand in a circle with hands joined.

## Chapter 7

# MEDITATION

It is the practice of concentrating on an object, word, or idea to clear the mind, relax the body, and achieve a state of heightened awareness and enlightment. Meditation has been a feature of many religions, but it can also serve as a practical, calming therapy. It cuts off the sensory input, halts the demands of the brain, and gives the mind a chance to rest. Research projects have shown that meditation can induce relaxation, lower blood pressure, reduce the body's metabolic rate and ameliorate many stress related disorders. It is one of the greatest methods to unwind, relax the mind and trigger the body's own natural relaxation response. It is not necessary to follow the teachings of a guru or mystic to benefit from meditation.

Try a simple form of meditating; find a quiet place and a comfortable sitting position that keeps your back straight. Close your eyes and concentrate on an image (a flame or flower) or on a sound or word (mantra) that will help clear your head of any extraneous thoughts. Breathe deeply and rhythmically, focussing attention on the chosen object or sound for 20 minutes.

There are various forms of meditation; some like Mantra meditation, Tatraka and Zazen meditation are quite popular, both in India and abroad. All methods of meditation are based on the principle of mind control, though they may use slightly different techniques. One can opt for any of the methods depending on the comfort level.

## Zazen Meditation

This is a very simple technique and with practice you can use it anywhere, whether you are at work, on a journey or at home.

- ❑ Choose your relaxation position and concentrate on your breathing, making it deep and even.

- Next, empty your mind of everything but your breathing. Concentrate on the sensations of your ribs and stomach moving in and out.
- To prevent your mind from wandering, you may find it useful to count up to ten as you breathe: inhale, exhale 'one'; inhale, exhale 'two'; and so on. Once you reach 'ten', start at 'one' once more.
- As you count, fix your mind on one particular aspect of the breathing process, your stomach, for example, or your breastbone, to the exclusion of all else.
- If your mind begins to wander, just start concentrating and counting again. The more you practise the less often you will find that this is necessary.

## Mantra Meditation

Transcendental gurus believe that only a guru can give a mantra, but others believe that a mantra is just as effective if chosen by the individual concerned. Your mantra should be a word that has no relevance or meaning. Just 'Om' is a good mantra. If a particular mantra does not appear to be effective after a few tries, choose a different word.

- Relax in your chosen position, eyes closed.
- Empty your mind and repeat your mantra as you breathe. Keep a steady rhythm.
- Ignore all thoughts that enter your mind. If you cannot and the rhythm of the mantra breaks down, just start again.

## Trataka Meditation

The trataka, or object, is simply used as a device for focussing concentration, because so many people find it easiest to concentrate on a physical object outside and apart from themselves rather than on a word.

- Choose a small object – it is traditional to choose a candle, partly because it is easy to concentrate on a light, which leaves an after image in the eye; but any small object will do: a crystal, for example, or a shell, a stone or a ball.

- ❑ Place your chosen object at a comfortable distance from the eye – normally a few feet away. The object should either be at eye level or just below it, because the eye muscles quickly tire if they are forced to look upwards for any length of time.
- ❑ Relax and breathe evenly and deeply. Look at the object and concentrate on it; feel its presence, focus on its shape, texture, weight and smell and sense its energy. Let these sensations float through your mind. Do not force them, though the process is completely passive one involving 'seeing', not an intellectual exercise.

As for the other methods, if your mind wanders, just start to concentrate on the object again. With practise, this will happen less frequently.

Chapter 8

# HYPNOTHERAPY

Hypnotherapy has been proved to solve a wide range of physical and psychological problems like asthma, eczema, irritable bowel syndrome and high blood pressure. Self hypnosis is easy to learn and effective. It is important to know that self-hypnosis takes time and effort. You will have to set aside some time every day to work on your techniques in order to realise the positive changes. Those who are self-motivated and determined to make things better achieve the best results.

## How Does Hypnotism Work

The brain is divided into two parts, the conscious mind and the sub conscious mind. The conscious mind controls and evaluates the world outside and sends messages and commands to the subconscious. The subconscious mind is similar to a computer; it has no critical faculty and accepts everything that is told by the conscious mind as a fact, even if it is not a fact. Once an idea is implanted in the subconscious mind though, the conscious mind has extreme difficulty in over riding it.

Self-hypnotism is a way of safely bypassing the conscious mind and reaching the subconscious mind. Self-hypnotism thus becomes an excellent way of combating stress related symptoms and of increasing the body's ability to relax and cope, mentally and physically.

## Guidelines for Success

To maximise the chance of success, any new ideas introduced to the subconscious should be –

- Genuine.
- Simple and positive.
- Use the present tense even if it sounds odd.

- ❑ Make sure that the idea refers to an action and not to an ability.
- ❑ Only try to implant one or two new ideas at a time.

## How to Self-hypnotise

Before attempting to achieve a light hypnotic trance, you must relax physically and try to convince yourself that you can hypnotise yourself. Remember that it is impossible to be hypnotised unless you consciously want this to happen.

A comfortable chair in a quiet room, and remember to take the telephone off the hook to prevent interruptions. Initially the session should be for about 20 – 30 minutes, but as your skill at entering the trance increases, you may wish to shorten them to 10 or 15 minutes.

The first step is to relax the body. Sit or lie down somewhere comfortable and close your eyes. Once you are completely relaxed, it is time to induce the hypnotic state. There are three methods of doing so.

### Eye fixation technique

This technique aims to induce the hypnotic state by developing a sense of fatigue and heaviness in the eye muscles and eyelids.

Look ahead, locate a spot above your line of sight and stare at it. Focus all your attention on that spot. As you blink or stare, your eyelids will begin to feel heavy. Allow them to droop, after a while. You breathing will slow to an even pace.

### Relaxation method

This method incorporates relaxed breathing, suggestions of calm, and muscle relaxation, to induce a peaceful trance state.

Close your eyes and focus on your breathing. Notice the rise and fall of your ribcage. Focus on the rest of your body, scanning it from head to toe for tensions of any kind. Allow tensions to leave your body and muscles to ease as you exhale.

Allow your relaxation to deepen, allowing the comfort you feel to sweep gently through your body.

### Staircase induction

Imagine yourself at the top of a beautiful staircase; examine it in detail in your mind. Decide on the place it leads to and imagine the most beautiful spot you would like it to be.

Count yourself down the steps from one to twenty, your mind becoming more relaxed and at ease with every step you take. Once you reach the bottom, explore it using all your senses. Find somewhere comfortable to sit in this scene, and relax.

Bring yourself out of the trance by counting backwards from three to one and then opening your eyes.

## Precautions

- Avoid self-hypnosis if you have a history of epilepsy. There is a slim chance that it may induce a fit.
- Never practice self-hypnosis when involved in any activity requiring you to be alert, for instance driving.
- If you intend to drive after self-hypnotic session, ensure that you are feeling fully alert.
- Psychotic and mentally unstable people should never attempt self-hypnosis.

*Chapter* **9**

# YOGA

In your fast-paced 20th Century existence, stress and tension continually appear on the horizon. Stress and tension are frequently thought to be the results of external situations. The yogi views this differently. Stress and tension are creations of your own mind. No external situation causes you to get upset or angry. Your mind does.

If you can be objective, think about things you like, or things that affect you in a certain way, for example, music. Some music you may really like. Someone else may think that this same music is horrible and that some other music, which you can't stand, is absolutely wonderful. You both hear the same music, made by the same vibrations. Is it the music, which makes you feel good or bad, or is it what your mind does with the sound vibrations after they enter your ears? Obviously, it's your mind.

The same is true with other external stimuli, which affect us in different ways, creating stress and tension. The bottom line is how our minds filter these stimuli. Some yoga tools help to change our perspective on the things that "create" stress and tension thereby helping you to cope better with everyday life.

The yogi sees your normal consciousness existing on three levels, the instinctive, the rational and the intuitive. The instinctive level is a very primal level, which deals with survival and happens "automatically"; it doesn't require any logic or reasoning. The rational level does involve thinking; it uses logic in solving your day-to-day problems. The intuitive level is yet a higher level of consciousness. Although we think we function best at the rational level, our optimum performance is on the intuitive level. Unfortunately, most people confuse emotionally generated thoughts and feelings with intuition. Through meditation, pranayama (yoga breathing exercises), relaxation techniques and yogic postures you can slowly open up your intuitive sphere, develop sensitivity and more inner awareness.

Yoga has been practised for thousands of years throughout the Indian sub-continent and is one of the six orthodox systems of Indian philosophy. Patanjali, the great sage, outlined the basic principles more than 2,000 years ago. According to him, there are eight stages in the quest for spiritual realisation-

| | |
|---|---|
| Yama | universal moral principles including non-violence, chastity, truthfulness, and absence of greed. |
| Niyama | purification of self through discipline and study. |
| Asanas | the postures of yoga. |
| Pranayama | the breathing techniques of yoga. |
| Pratyahara | freeing the mind from the domination of the senses and of the distractions of the outside world. |
| Dharana | deep concentration. |
| Dhyana | meditation |
| Samadhi | the state in which the soul is supreme. |

For a contented life you need a harmonious balance between your body, soul and mind, according to yoga philosophy. The pressures of modern society make it difficult to maintain equilibrium. Yoga is particularly beneficial in combating stress and stress related illnesses as it helps both the mind and the body.

By regular practice of the asanas, the body is strengthened and concentration is also improved. Doctors have accepted the benefits of yoga in lowering blood pressure, increasing body's strength and flexibility and helping to alleviate a wide range of problems including rheumatism, arthritis, back problems, menstrual disorders, migraine, and circulatory as well as digestive disorders.

Practising 'Suryà namaskar', and yogic dhyana, has immense effect on the mind.

Chapter 10

# MASSAGE

It's no secret that a good massage can help relax you or uncramp a muscle. More and more studies are confirming that just being touched regularly can boost mental and physical powers and improve quality of life for just about everyone – sick and well, young and old alike. We now know that human beings who don't get touched enough simply don't thrive, physically or emotionally.

Less well-known – but increasingly documented even by mainstream researchers – are all the ways a little "hands-on" can help speed healing, improve thinking skills, and even help relieve pain and other chronic ailments. Study after study is showing that regular massage can even improve your overall health, whether you measure health by how many cups of coffee you drink, how many trips you make to the doctor, how many social occasions you attend, or whatever.

## Massage Basics

Massage can make you feel better because it seems to affect almost everything your body does. Massage may improve circulation, bust stress, relieve pain, lower heart rate and blood pressure, reduce swelling, strengthen muscles, promote healing, restore motion to joints, and accelerate basic bodily functions (such as how fast you get rid of wastes).

Credible studies are starting to show that massage may even enhance immune response, perhaps by encouraging the brain to release fewer stress hormones and/or more natural painkillers into the bloodstream.

When most people think of massage, they're thinking of some version of Swedish massage. This technique – developed in the early 19th century by a gymnastics instructor who cured himself of an elbow problem by tapping on it – was first brought to the United States in the 1850s, where today it's the most popular massage technique.

But massage is actually a much broader term. It's defined as "systematic manipulation of the soft tissues of the body" (such as muscle and connective tissue). Manipulation can mean any combination of rubbing, kneading, slapping, tapping, rolling, pressing, or jostling, as long as the goal is to make you feel better.

Close to one hundred different techniques fit this definition of massage, most of which were developed in the past 20 years. Many massage therapists use a variety of these techniques.

## Tips to Make the Most of Massage

- ❑ You don't need to let common myths and fears stress you out about the massage that's supposed to relax you. Keeping the following points in mind can help
- ❑ Be sure that you feel comfortable with your therapist. Getting touched is fairly personal, and you should feel safe in the process.
- ❑ Let the therapist know what you want – or ask for help deciding. Is your main goal to relax, or is it to relieve a specific injury or pain? How heavy or light should the pressure be?
- ❑ Ask the therapist to avoid sensitive areas. If your right shin is tender, there's no reason it has to be massaged (unless you and the therapist think a massage may help heal it). And if you're embarrassed to have anyone touch your neck or right knee or whatever, speak up. Well-trained, professional massage therapists should have a very good sense of clients' personal boundaries and will take these issues quite seriously.
- ❑ Take off only the clothes you feel comfortable taking off.
- ❑ Prepare to relax. It's usually a good idea to avoid eating a heavy meal right before a massage. Some people find it helps to take a shower or bath right before the massage.

- ❑ Speak up if something hurts or tickles. Sometimes a massage can cause temporary discomfort, especially if it involves working on sore, damaged, or tense areas. You may even feel sore in these areas for a day or two after a massage, just like underused muscles can feel sore after unfamiliar exercise.
- ❑ Speak up if you're sensitive to the aroma of the oil or just can't stand that soporific music in the background. You're the client.
- ❑ Remember, though, that speaking up has its limits. Focus on your breathing and the soothing hands, the soothing oils, and the relaxing music.
- ❑ Leave time to savour the results. Jumping back into your business suit and hailing a taxi may be unavoidable, but ideally you should leave yourself a few minutes to enjoy. Meanwhile, drink lots of water, which supposedly keeps the circulation flowing (and is actually a good idea for everyone, as long as you don't have a problem with congestive heart failure).

## Massage: Benefits and Possible Harm

While it is helpful to know what benefits can be reaped from massage therapy, it is equally as important to be aware of the possible harm that may come about.

### Benefits

Besides helping you relax, soothing sore muscles, reducing some kinds of swelling, and improving general well-being, massage therapy of one sort or another may also help with hypertension, burns, chronic pain (including from arthritis, backaches, and migraines), rashes and other skin conditions, addictions, depression, stress and pain of labour, asthma, and attention deficit hyperactivity disorder (ADHD).

It can also alleviate depression and boost self-esteem in people with eating disorders; improve growth and development in premature babies; reduce pain and water retention in women with premenstrual syndrome (PMS); raise blood sugar levels in kids with diabetes; and possibly even boost immune function in people with HIV or cancer.

## Possible harm

Massage strikes a lot of people as harmless, but it's actually a powerful tool (if it weren't, how could it help all those ailments?). And it follows that a procedure that has so much power to do good can also – if used inappropriately – sometimes have the power to cause damage. This potential for harm is all the more reason to see a therapist who knows what he's doing – and we don't just mean knows how to give a good back rub. A qualified therapist not only knows a good deal about the human body, how it works, and what can go wrong with it, but also is willing to tell you when massage is inappropriate or dangerous.

If you have a serious or chronic illness, never use massage without first consulting a doctor. You should also generally avoid using massage on inflamed, burned, or otherwise injured areas. And because massage works by promoting blood flow, it can potentially spread certain problems throughout your body. You should almost always avoid massage therapy if you have an infection, cancer, swelling (oedema), or a blood clot (except under the supervision of a highly skilled physician). People with high blood pressure, an enlarged liver or spleen, or peptic ulcers should also avoid abdominal massages. And pregnant women should stick to well-trained, professional massage therapists who are familiar with pregnancy massage.

# Chapter 11

# T'AI CHI CH'UAN

T'ai chi chuan – T'ai chi for short – is an ancient Chinese technique that applies the principle of Taoist philosophy to the art of movement. The basis of Taoist philosophy is the search for natural balance and harmony in all things. It is based on the principle of 'yin' and 'yang', and the idea that to find a personal harmony we need to accept what is – the natural order of the universe and use this, rather than resisting it, to achieve our goals. In this way we reaming in balance both within the outside world and ourselves.

T'ai chi has been described as 'meditation in motion'; each movement or exercise has a symbolic interpretation placed upon the psychological element involved. It aims to expand our consciousness of ourselves as a mental and physical whole and realise the power that we have within us.

A lot of people claim that Tai Chi may provide the same cardiovascular benefits as strenuous exercise without putting the same strain on the heart — and evidence for these claims is starting to roll in. Tai Chi may also reduce symptoms of Parkinson's disease and help prevent falls in the elderly. A few studies have already shown that Tai Chi can improve breathing, reduce stress, lower blood pressure, and improve balance — although whether it can do these things any better than other techniques remains to be seen.

## Postures

T'ai chi consists of a number of basic posture called 'forms' and a large and varied collection of exercises. Each form is a complicated series of postures that are all linked to give one flowing movement. All the movements are circular and aim to develop muscular control, rather than muscular bulk. In order to learn these, it is best to attend a few classes and then to practice them at home.

As one follows the forms, the body will become relaxed. The mind also becomes relaxed as it concentrates on the flow of relaxed movements. Throughout each exercise the body should be relaxed and the movements slow and the mind centred inwards to feel the flow of energy. Try to forget the presence of time.

Chapter 12

# AROMA THERAPY

Aromatherapy means "treatment using scents". It is a holistic treatment of caring for the body with pleasant smelling botanical oils such as rose, lemon, lavender and peppermint. The essential oils are added to the bath or massaged into the skin, inhaled directly or diffused to scent an entire room. Aromatherapy is used for the relief of pain, care for the skin, alleviate tension and fatigue and invigorate the entire body. Essential oils can affect the mood, alleviate fatigue, reduce anxiety and promote relaxation. When inhaled, they work on the brain and nervous system through stimulation of the olfactory nerves.

The essential oils are aromatic essences extracted from plants, flowers, trees, fruits, bark, grasses and seeds with distinctive therapeutic, psychological, and physiological properties, which improve and prevent illness. There are about 150 essential oils. Most of these oils have antiseptic properties; some are antiviral, anti-inflammatory, pain relieving, antidepressant and expectorant. Essential oils have other benefits like stimulation, relaxation, digestion improvement, and diuretic properties. To get the maximum benefit from essential oils, it should be made from natural, pure raw materials. Synthetically made oils do not work. Aromatherapy is one of the fastest growing fields in alternative medicine.

It is widely used at home, clinics and hospitals for a variety of applications such as pain relief for women in labour pain, relieving pain caused by the side effects of the chemotherapy undergone by the cancer patients, and rehabilitation of cardiac patients. Aromatherapy is already slowly getting into the mainstream. In Japan, engineers are incorporating aroma systems into new buildings. In one such application, the scent of lavender and rosemary is pumped into the customer area to calm down the waiting customers, while the perfumes from lemon and eucalyptus is used in the bank teller counters to keep the staff alert. Four drops of camomile, with four drops of marjoram and two drops of sandalwood added to the bath can relieve tension.

## How Does Aromatherapy Work

Essential oils stimulate the powerful sense of smell. It is known that smell has a significant impact on how we feel. In dealing with patients who have lost the sense of smell, doctors have found that a life without fragrance can lead to high incidence of psychiatric problems such as anxiety and depression. We have the capability to distinguish 10,000 different smells. It is believed that smells enter through cilia (the fine hairs lining the nose) to the limbic system, the part of the brain that controls our moods, emotions, memory and learning. Studies with brain wave frequency have shown that smelling lavender increases alpha waves in the back of the head, which are associated with relaxation.

Fragrance of Jasmine increases beta waves in the front of the head, which are associated with a more alert state. Scientific studies have also shown that essential oils contain chemical components that can exert specific effects on the mind and body.

## Some Symptoms and Effective Essential Oils

| | |
|---|---|
| **Tension** | bergamot; camomile; marjoram; neroli; sandalwood; camphor; jasmine. |
| **Colic** | marjoram; clary sage; juniper. |
| **Indigestion** | bergamot; fennel; lemon; peppermint. |

| | |
|---|---|
| **Diarrhoea** | eucalyptus; juniper; neroli; sandalwood. |
| **Muscular aches and pains** | eucalyptus; rosemary; sage. |
| **Depression** | bergamot; geranium; jasmine; neroli; rose; ylang ylang. |
| **Insomnia** | camphor; camomile; jasmine; marjoram; neroli. |
| **Headaches** | cardamom; lavender; marjoram; peppermint; rose. |

Each essential oil contains as much as 100 chemical components, which together exert a strong effect on the whole person. Depending on which component is predominating in an oil, the oils act differently. For example, some oils are relaxing, some soothes you down, some relieves your pain, etc. Then there are oils such as lemon and lavender, which adapt to what your body needs, and adapt to that situation. (These are called "adaptogenic"). The mechanism in which these essential oils act on us is not very well understood. What is understood is that they affect our mind and emotions. They leave no harmful residues. They enter into the body either by absorption or inhalation.

A fragrance company in Japan conducted studies to determine the effects of smell on people. They have pumped different fragrances in an area where a number of keyboard entry operators were stationed and monitored the number of mistakes made as a function of the smell in the air. The results were as follows:

- When exposed to lavender oil fragrance (a relaxant), the keyboard typing errors dropped 20 percent.
- When exposed to jasmine (an uplifting fragrance), the errors dropped 33 percent. When exposed to lemon fragrance (a sharp, refreshing stimulant), the mistakes fell by a whopping 54 percent!

There are many techniques that have been found to be effective in promoting relaxation and work as stress relievers. These are just a few of them. There are so many types of relaxation techniques that one single book cannot contain them. One can opt for the technique that is most suitable or device a new one to suit himself by combining two or more techniques.

Chapter 13

# COLOUR THERAPY

## What is Colour Therapy

This form of therapy has been practised as far back in time as the ancient Indian and Egyptian civilizations. In ancient Egypt, people often immersed themselves in vats of coloured pigment as a curative measure. There were great halls with coloured glass panels or windows where people would stand and be bathed in the light that filtered in. The light streaming in through the stained glass in European churches clearly have a soothing effect. The sun's rays are known to have almost magical healing qualities and these rays passed through a spectrum, produced colours that were used to cure illnesses and injuries. Colour therapy has always been one of the main weapons employed against disease by Ayurvedic practitioners.

Research results from New England, in the United States, have shown that colour has an effect on blood pressure: after 30 minutes of exposure to blue light, blood pressure dropped: after the same time in red light, blood pressure rose. Many people could lower their blood pressure for a moment or two just by visualizing the colour blue.

## Benefits of Colour Therapy

- Colour has an effect on the mental and physical make-up of an individual.
- Bright colours are known to add colour to a person's life.
- Colour therapy has helped in anti-ageing process.
- Colour therapy works in spiritual healing.
- Diseases like arthritis and tuberculosis and skin diseases are known to be cured by this form of alternative healing.

## Colours and Their Effects

### Red

Stimulating, aggressive, strengthens will power and stimulates vitality. This colour helps to loosen stiffness and restraints. It stimulates the release of adrenaline in the bloodstream and causes haemoglobin to multiply. Hence, it results in greater strength and energy and is good for treating anaemia and other blood-related conditions. Red can also make you feel warmer, reducing pain that comes from the cold. Helpful in lethargy and depression, but use with caution, since this colour can be very powerful; always follow with exposure to blue to create harmony. An excess of red can make a person agitated and aggressive. While it may excite sexual passion, it can also lead to anger and destructive behaviour. People who have heart trouble or a nervous disposition should be careful before they use this colour.

### Orange

Warm, suggests a sense of well-being and restores vitality. Orange is also a colour of energy. It is used to increase immunity, sexual potency; it helps in all digestive ailments, chest and kidney diseases. It is used to treat negative feelings, insecurity, inertia, lassitude, odd aches and pains and muscular cramps. Orange has a gentle warming effect if used lightly. Orange, like red should not be used for too long. It is not a good colour for 'nervy' people or people who get easily agitated.

### Yellow

Powerful and mentally stimulating, it helps to cure depression, skin problems and mental lethargy... Yellow stimulates the intellect and has a generally cheering effect. It has been found useful in facilitating the digestive process. However, like red and orange, it is not recommended for people experiencing great stress. Over stimulation could result in exhaustion and depression.

### Green

Gives a sense of proportion and balance, restoring the body's natural harmony. Used to treat tension (especially

headaches), stress, moodiness and over-emotional behaviour. Green helps to calm frazzled nerves and is good for people with heart conditions. It stimulates growth and therefore helps to heal broken bones and facilitates the regrowth of tissue. It is recommended for pregnant women to create a serene atmosphere. However, too much green can bring on a sense of lethargy as the person settles into a state of tranquillity almost approaching stagnation. A person tends to become complacent, as he does not feel a sense of challenge or a need to strive towards any goal.

## Lavender

The colour lavender represents equilibrium; it helps in spiritual healing. It is used as a tranquilliser and aids sleep. It is a colour of replenishing and rebuilding. It is like a tonic for the body. Too much will make you very tired and disoriented.

## White

This colour represents purity. It purifies the body on the highest levels. It brings peace and comfort and is the best reliever of pain.

## Silver

Silver is the colour of peace and persistence. It is a purging colour and is very good for removing unwanted diseases and troubles from the body. It is best for cancer of tissue and blood.

## Gold

Gold is the strongest colour and helps cure almost all illness. It is so strong that most people are unable to tolerate it and need to be conditioned to it gradually and over a period of time. Gold strengthens all fields of the body and spirit.

## Black

Black is a colour that is not used very often because overexposure can leave one looking tired and haggard. Indian climatic conditions are not ideal for this colour.

### Blue
Calming, relaxing and cleansing; symbolises love and truth. Helpful in encouraging relaxation, especially when feeling irritable, jumpy or aggressive.

### Indigo
Cool and clarifying, restores a balance between the individual and the outside world. Used to treat obsessions and emotional instability.

### Violet
Harmonises the body, mind and spirit. As ultra-violet, this colour is used in conventional western medicine to treat skin conditions and to restore the body's natural balance of salts. Use at home to treat insomnia, over-sensitivity and tension.

### Blue-green
These shades are particularly useful in promoting relaxation and the release of tension.

### Pink
Traditionally, the colour of love. Use it to create a feeling of warmth coupled with energy.

### Peach-apricot
Warm and relaxing; ideal when you feel physically exhausted.

## How to Use Colour Therapy
Colour therapy can be practised in the following ways-

### At home
- ❑ Coloured light bulbs and coloured glass windows.
- ❑ When decorating, use earth colours like peaches, pinks, greens and warm blues.
- ❑ Never decorate a sunless room in a dark or cold colour - doing so will make the walls crowd in and produce a feeling of claustrophobia.
- ❑ Use plants and flowers to add colour and life to a drab room.

- ❑ Add food colouring to your bath water – green and blue to relax, or orange and red to stimulate.
- ❑ Use vivid coloured cushions to brighten a dull room.
- ❑ Try to make sure that at least one room in your house has a décor that is relaxing and soothing – make use of this space when you feel depressed.
- ❑ Solarized water can be used as a healing tonic. In this method, purified water is filled in a clear container of the prescribed colour and left out in the sun for a couple of hours. The sun's rays filter through the coloured glass.

## Wearing the colours

- ❑ Choose your clothes according to their colour, to enhance or change your mood.
- ❑ Either throw out drab, washed-out clothes or dye them another colour.
- ❑ Liven up clothes with a colourful scarf, a tie, a belt or jewellery.
- ❑ Experiment with different colours. Withdrawn, shy people often wear greys and browns: add a striking and contrasting scarf or shirt.
- ❑ Irritable, noisy people tend to use red, black and orange: contrast with turquoise, blue and green.
- ❑ Cold, over-controlled people generally wear blues, greys and blacks: warm your outlook with pinks, peaches and apricot.

## Using colours creatively

- ❑ Eat and drink foods and liquids of the colours you wish to emphasize. If you wish to become more outgoing, for example, try eating oranges and drinking orange or carrot juice. Solarising the drinking water will also help.
- ❑ Swathe your body in an appropriate colour by fitting a coloured light bulb to a lamp.
- ❑ Practise visualising the colour that you need to change or enhance your mood. Most people find this difficult at first, but succeed with practice.

Try what is called 'colour breathing': either bathe yourself and the room in the colour of your choice, or visualise the colour, then relax and breathe deeply, holding your breath for a few seconds while you concentrate on the colour filling your body. Breathe out and repeat 3 or 4 times, then relax. Repeat this exercise three times a week.

## Healing Power of Prayers

In Hindi movies whenever anyone is critically ill the doctor advises his kin to pray for the recovery of the patient. Most of us do not take this advice seriously but now it has been proved that there is a definite relation between prayers and healing. This is also the reason that many REIKI believers organise group healing and prayer sessions for those combating serious ailments.

The National Institute of Health, USA reviewed more than 250 studies published since the 19th century and discovered a positive connection between prayer and healing for nearly every kind of cancer, cardiovascular disease, hypertension, colitis, enteritis and even diabetes. It has also been found that the patients who are prayed for by friends, family or prayer groups, even when they are located half way around the earth, are likely to recover faster from illnesses than those who have nobody praying for them.

Says Dr. Harold G. Koenig, Director of the Programme on Religion, Ageing and Health at Duke University Medical Centre in Durham, North Carolina, USA – "We're beginning to see that having faith in God, a higher power that listens, cares and responds, can be a very powerful force in healing. All the evidence says that prayer does have an impact."

For complete and holistic health, therefore, it is essential that a part of your daily schedule should be spent in praying. Whichever be the religion you follow, communion with God will bring peace and health to you.

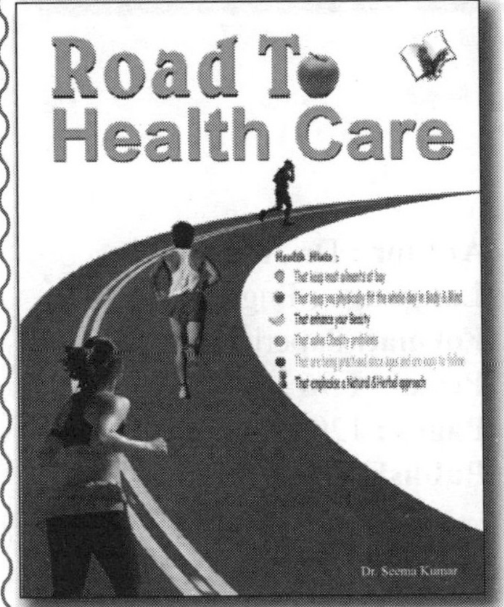


**Author :** Dr. Seema Kumar
**Language :** English
**Format:** Paperback
**Price :** ₹ 175
**Pages :** 176
**Publisher: V&S Publishers**

With ever-rising ground, water and atmospheric pollution, every other day one hears the name of a new disease. Ever since man began drifting away from Nature, he is falling into the trap of a materialistic lifestyle that has desensitised him. Today, we breathe air thick with exhaust fumes, eat processed junk food that has no nutritive value, drink toxic carbonated beverages and lead sedentary lives. All of this ensures that we are plagued with different kinds of problems at regular intervals.

This book shows you how to go back to Mother Nature to beat even the most troublesome and chronic ailments. With natural preventive measures that emphasise diet, exercise and herbal remedies, there are no fears of obnoxious side effects.

Whatever be your problem – diabetes, blood pressure, asthma, acne, menopause, obesity, stomach ailments, premature ageing or general complaints – this book shows you a safe, natural and enjoyable means to overcome it. Most of the ingredients mentioned in the book are the kind available in home gardens or off the kitchen shelf.

The book also includes hints for different stages in life. A separate section deals with varied problems in a woman's life through adolescence, pregnancy, lactation, menopause and general ailments.

Once you have read this book from cover to cover, you need not rush to the doctor every now and then, but will be able to take care of your own and your family's health yourself.

## DIABETES CONTROL IN YOUR HANDS

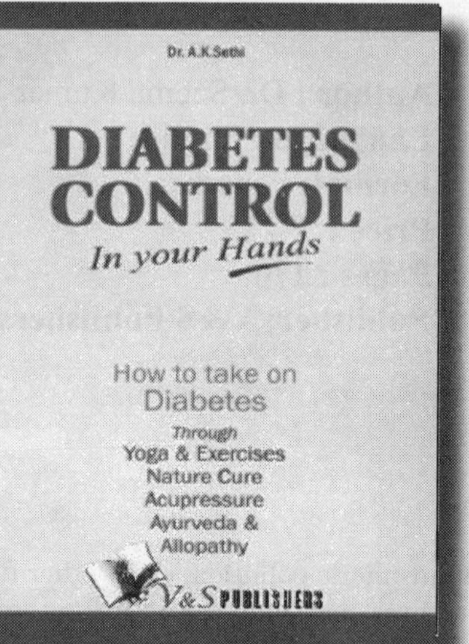


**Author :** Dr. A.K. Sethi
**Language :** English
**Format:** Paperback
**Price :** ₹ 96
**Pages :** 120
**Publisher: V&S Publishers**

Take on Diabetes through Diet-control, Yoga & Exercise, Nature Cure, Acupressure, Ayurveda and Allopathy.

Since diabetes cannot be cured, the only way to deal with it is to learn how to control it. With this clear objective in view, the book offers a complete guide on the ways and means to go about it.

Where the book scores over others is that it does not just confine itself to Allopathic treatment but offers a complete controlling mechanism covering Ayurveda, Yoga, Nature Cure, Acupressure, Feng Shui through conventional and non-conventional ways.

This book is a must not only for those affected by diabetes, but everyone above forty who could run the risk of getting it.

**All books available at www.vspublishers.com**

## HEALING HEART DISEASE NATURALLY

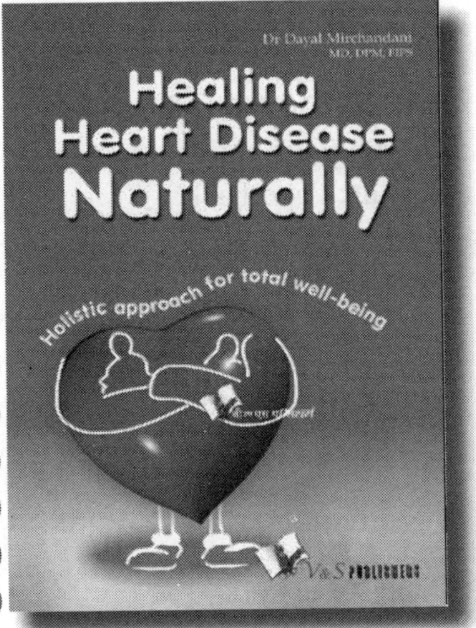


**Author :** Dr. Dayal Mirchandani
**Language :** English
**Format:** Paperback
**Price :** ₹ 96
**Pages :** 200
**Publisher: V&S Publishers**

Recent advances in the behavioural sciences have ensured that a variety of physical disorders can be healed using psychological techniques.

In fact, worldwide, mind-body healing is being increasingly used to treat chronic illnesses such as asthma, ulcerative colitis, rheumatoid arthritis and coronary artery disease with excellent results.

This book reveals the personality trait that puts you at highest risk and how to change it, how to use self-hypnosis and imagery in healing your heart, how to stop smoking permanently with little or no discomfort, how to find meaning and joy in life, besides other practical techniques to reverse heart disease.

## KEY TO STRESS-FREE LIVING

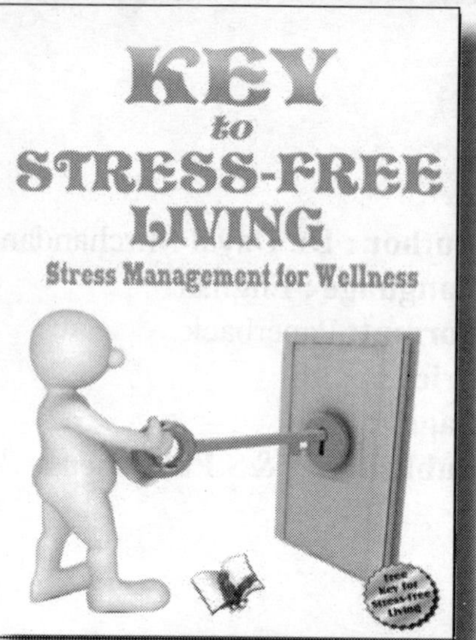


*Free Keychain*

**Author :** Dr. Jyotsna Codaty
**Language :** English
**Format:** Paperback
**Price :** ₹ 150
**Pages :** 136
**Publisher: V&S Publishers**

There are three primary aspects of life that contribute to promoting unhealthy stress which ultimately kills – inability to make decisions, feeling lack of control in life, and not having a plan or process in place to get to where you need to go. Spread over 18 chapters, this book has put together all the necessary materials to take control of your life, make wise decisions, and be proactive in taking care of things that typically stress you out. This book contains principles and ideas that will go a long way in reducing the stress that people have in this 21st century.

The fact that you are reading the blurb of a book on stress management, maybe out of sheer curiosity, signifies that you are trying to decipher if life could be made more meaningful and positive, no matter how contented or stressful life you are leading at the moment. This book is full of tips worth reading, especially given the author's credentials.

**All books available at www.vspublishers.com**

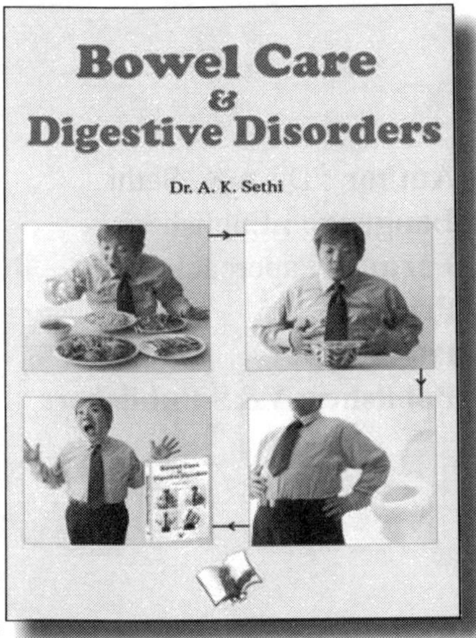


**Author :** Dr. A.K. Sethi
**Language :** English
**Format:** Paperback
**Price :** ₹ 135
**Pages :** 132
**Publisher: V&S Publishers**

Most people are shy about discussing Bowel care & Digestive Disorders, but few realize how important it is. The truth is that it needs utmost care and attention. The bowel has very few nervous leads- otherwise you would feel the digestion and bowel movement all day long. So, if you feel you have a digestive problem of sorts, you better attend to it immediately.

Most toxins enter our body through the digestive tract, along with our food and drinks. If we don't eat healthy, we tend to accumulate toxic wastes resulting in increased bowel transit time, and the wastes, instead of getting eliminated, stay put inside our body. These wastes, putrefy further and become a breeding ground for harmful bacteria and other parasites which in turn leads to more serious diseases and problems developing in the body.

This book is an authoritative reference source on bowel care and digestive disorders of various types. Written in a very convincing and captivating manner providing some anatomy lessons about the digestive tract, causes and symptoms of bowel disorders (constipation, diarrhea, etc.), the book lists proper diagnosis and treatment. It has been designed as an ideal self-help guide through yoga, meditation, ayurvedic treatment and alternative treatment methods like magneto therapy, acupressure, colour therapy, vastu, aromatherapy and music therapy to manage bowel disorders.

## HOW TO HAVE SOUND SLEEP

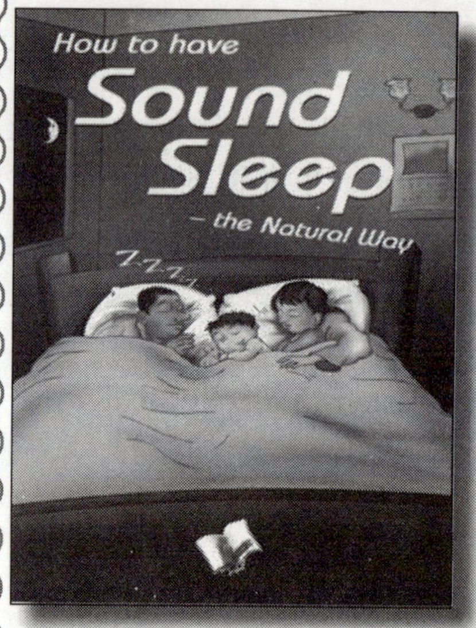


**Author :** Dr. A.K. Sethi
**Language :** English
**Format:** Paperback
**Price :** ₹ 135
**Pages :** 136
**Publisher: V&S Publishers**

Sleep Deprivation Can Make You Obese, Forgetful, Aged and Diseased for the Rest of Your Life!

Don't blame lifestyle for your disturbed sleep. Did you know that sleeping more or fewer than seven hours a day greatly impairs the production of thyroid and stress hormones. This impairment, in turn, not only affects the memory, immune system and metabolism etc., but also increases the risk of high blood sugar levels, hypertension (high blood pressure), weight gain, accelerated ageing, depression and increased risk of heart attack.

Researchers have also determined that sleeping adequately after a few days of disturbed sleep can very nearly erase any lingering sense of mental haziness and fatigue. In order to help you get a sound sleep and also to protect you from the need to take recourse to making up any lost sleep or disorder, the book details the importance, benefits, physiology and body reinvigoration of having sound sleep, untoward effects of sleep disorders and natural & non-conventional methods of managing it. Also explained in various chapters are advantages of proper exercise, yoga, naturopathy, acupressure, colour & music therapy, lifestyle changes etc., that enable waking up in the morning feeling fresh, fit and trim. A separate chapter is devoted to the Dos and Don'ts to highlight factors that contribute towards bringing sound sleep.

An indispensible book guaranteeing Sound Sleep to all readers every night!



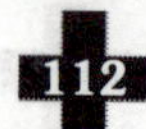